MEDICAL EDUCATION

MEDICAL EDUCATION

STELLA LOWRY, MB

Assistant editor, British Medical Journal

With an introduction by
SIR DAVID WEATHERALL, FRS

*Professor of medicine, Nuffield
Department of Clinical Medicine,
John Radcliffe Hospital, Oxford*

Published by the BMJ Publishing Group
Tavistock Square, London WC1H 9JR

First published 1993

British Library Cataloguing in Publication Data
A catalogue record for this book is available from the British Library

ISBN 0-7279-0780-8

The following picture sources are acknowledged:

Page 4, Format; page 12, Sally and Richard Greenhill; pages 22, 30, 41, University of Newcastle upon Tyne; page 48, St Bartholomew's Hospital; page 55, Homer Sykes/Impact; page 62, Sally and Richard Greenhill; page 69, Homer Sykes/Impact; page 72, Adam Rouilly (London) Ltd; page 78, BMA News Review; page 81, Neil Turner/Insight.

Typeset by Bedford Typesetters Limited, Bedford
Printed and bound in Great Britain by
Eyre & Spottiswoode Ltd, London and Margate

Acknowledgments

I thank the many people who helped in my research for this book. In particular, I thank Dr Angela Towle of the King's Fund Centre, London, for comment and advice at every stage.

Contents

Introduction

"Something is seriously wrong with medical education in Britain."
The pessimistic opening salvo which introduces this stimulating book
by Stella Lowry is based on impressions gleaned from conversations
with deans of teaching hospitals, the General Medical Council's recent
review of medical education, and a lengthy national consensus inquiry
organised by the King's Fund. It seems that there is widespread
agreement that our present medical school curricula are grossly
overcrowded with factual information and that our students are
inhibited from developing into creative, critical thinkers and
"problem solvers." There are, of course, problems even with these
distinguished sources of information. Much of the evidence on which
their conclusions are based is anecdotal, and none of them, at least to
my knowledge, has ever looked at a control group of graduates from
other fields; I doubt if any students worth their salt are ever satisfied
with a degree course. Those who take medical education seriously
have never been happy about what they are doing. Our present soul
searching is reminiscent of what George Pickering was saying 30 years
ago, and, for that matter, of Thomas Sydenham's views of medical
education in Oxford in the seventeenth century—one of his contem-
poraries recorded that Sydenham thought it better to send a man to
Oxford to be instructed in shoemaking than to learn how to practise
medicine. However, the fact that each generation of clinical teachers
seems to make a mess of things is certainly not a reason for
complacency.

One of the major frustrations for medical educationalists is that
there is no way of measuring the end result. The skills and attitudes

required for a good doctor are not something that can be acquired in a few years at medical school, nor can they be assessed by a final qualifying test or by any form of examination. If we were ever able to devise appropriate methods for assessing what we are trying to do we would have to look at our products 20 years or more after qualification. Furthermore, we are trying to design a course to prepare young people for activities which range from a full time career in basic science, through hospital medicine or general practice, to the directorship of a pharmaceutical company. And it is inappropriate to take undergraduate teaching out of the context of the overall training of doctors. It is no use developing a generation of creative, critical thinkers only for many of them to become disillusioned by a ridiculously long period of apprenticeship or the mind numbing requirements of some of our specialist examinations.

Another major problem for medical education is that it has to adapt itself to the constantly changing scene of clinical science and practice. Sitting through a recent selection committee for a consultant physician, at which the entire conversation revolved round purchasing and providing, and at which clinical practice, teaching, and research were rarely mentioned, I wondered whether our graduates of the future would be better prepared for their professional lives by spending their postgraduate years in a business management college rather than striving to obtain a diploma from one of the medical royal colleges, let alone developing clinical and pastoral skills. It is clear that we cannot go on adding more and more to our courses. Most medical schools have simply grafted on each new development as it has come along; molecular biology, communication skills, ethics, and business management are just a few of the dishes that have been added to an overly rich diet in recent years. No wonder many of our young doctors are not, to borrow one of CP Snow's favourite academic labels, graduating in a state of "smiling eupepsia."

There is good sense in thinking about a "core" curriculum—if nothing else it is good self discipline for teachers and will provide students with a much clearer idea of what is expected of them. But it will not be easy to construct, as is already apparent from the efforts of the General Medical Council. And we shall have to design a series of stimulating options round the core, courses which offer a glimpse of the breadth and excitement of the many and varied facets of medicine. And, above all, we shall have to address our major national disgrace, the preregistration year. We have much to learn from the American training programmes for house staff.

One of the great attractions of medicine as a profession is the enormous diversity of careers that it offers. It follows, therefore, that medical education should be equally varied. There is no one way to educate a doctor. The exciting new programmes at Harvard and McMaster universities, or more conventional approaches still to be found in some of the older (but not yet completely ossified) British universities, all have their place. What excites students is not so much the content of the course but the quality and enthusiasm of their teachers. I hope that all those interested and involved in medical education will read Stella Lowry's excellent book and think again about what they are trying to do. But although I agree with most of what Dr Lowry has to say I remain to be convinced that there is a crisis in medical education; there will only be a genuine crisis when those who teach medical students are convinced that they have got it right.

D J WEATHERALL

What's wrong with medical education in Britain?

Something is seriously wrong with medical education in Britain. Professor Lesley Rees, dean of St Bartholomew's Hospital Medical College, London, recalls with horror the transformation of eager, motivated school leavers into narrow minded, disillusioned medical graduates. "Immediately I became subdean at Barts there was a great stamping of feet into my office, with complaints about everything. I cannot remember half of them, but it was a depressing experience to hear young men and women complaining of all the inadequacies that they perceived in the educational process that they had been through for five years." The General Medical Council admits that the traditional medical course is stifling students: "Imagination and curiosity are soon dulled and learning patterns quickly adapt to the need to absorb knowledge, often at a superficial level."[1] A recent national consensus inquiry organised by the King's Fund confirmed that such worries about the undergraduate medical curriculum are widespread: "There is widespread agreement that present curricula are grossly overcrowded with factual information which soon becomes out of date and inhibits students from developing into creative critical thinkers and problem solvers."[2]

Faulty approach to medical education?

This crisis in medical education is part of a wider crisis in medicine. Data from UCCA (Universities' Central Council on Admissions) confirm that fewer people are applying to study medicine despite large increases in applications for tertiary education as a whole. Increasing

1

numbers of doctors are admitting to being stressed and disillusioned by their jobs,[3 4] many regretting their choice of career.[5] The *Doctors to Be* series on BBC television (following medical students through their course at St Mary's Hospital Medical School, London) provided ample evidence of this disenchantment: "It could have been such a wonderful thing to be a doctor—but it's not. It's just a disaster."[6] The undergraduate medical course is often identified as contributing to this demoralisation by deadening the students' initial enthusiasm and failing to prepare them adequately for the realities of professional life.[7]

Is this criticism justified, and can we reverse some of the recent trends by changing our approach to medical education?

The traditional British medical course

The traditional British medical course was divided into three parts. The first part lasted one year and consisted of the premedical sciences of chemistry, physics, and biology (1st MB). The 2nd MB course occupied two years, during which the preclinical sciences of biochemistry, anatomy, and physiology were studied. The clinical course occupied the final three years and led to the qualification MB, BS (bachelor of medicine and surgery).

Few schools still offer a premedical course, and the usual medical course now occupies five years and is equivalent to the 2nd and 3rd MBs.

Most schools provide an opportunity for selected students to spend an additional intercalated year studying for the degree of bachelor of science (BSc) or bachelor of medical science (BMedSci) during the course, and about a fifth of medical students take up this option. Some schools now offer a BMedSci as a routine part of the medical course for all of their students.

Traditionally, medical students spend their preclinical years in the medical schools, where they are taught by university staff who are rarely medically qualified. The clinical teaching has, however, always been based in NHS hospitals, where the clinical academic staff hold honorary NHS appointments. Thus the Department of Health has an interest, if little direct control, in the process of medical education.

On completion of the undergraduate course a doctor obtains provisional registration with the GMC but can practise independently only after a further year of apprenticeship in approved posts. This preregistration year provides "general clinical training," which combines with the undergraduate course to form what is known as "basic medical education." Traditionally a doctor who had completed basic medical education and obtained full registration could work as an independent medical practitioner.

In this book I shall explore some of the most important themes in medical education. During my researches I have visited medical schools in Britain and abroad and have discussed the current problems and possible solutions with medical students, academic teaching staff, deans, NHS doctors, professional educationalists, people who have already introduced innovative schemes into medical courses, and representatives of official bodies like the GMC and the BMA. I have learnt a lot about how the current problems are perceived and where possible solutions might lie.

I now want to introduce some of the basic principles, debunk a few myths, highlight innovative schemes, and explain some of the educational jargon. I am not writing for the professional medical educators but for the vast majority of doctors for whom teaching is part of their daily lives but who are too often excluded from the current debates. I shall concentrate on basic medical education (the undergraduate course and the preregistration year), though I realise that medical education is an ongoing, ideally lifelong activity and that any end point is arbitrary.

What are the problems?

The problems in medical education permeate every aspect of the system. Even before students arrive at medical school the problems have started. In recent years there has been a steady drop in the number of people applying to study medicine, despite an increasing number of applicants for other university courses. Overall there are only two applicants for each place in British medical schools each year. Possible explanations include the recent publicity given to the junior doctors' hours of work campaign, recognition that many doctors regret their choice of careers,[5] and changes in the public's attitude to the medical profession, with some loss of the traditional awe associated with being a doctor. There has also been a reduction in the relative earning power of doctors compared with other professionals, and the student loan scheme and the recession are additional financial disincentives for people contemplating a long university course with short holidays in which they cannot hope to supplement their incomes by taking holiday jobs.

Then there are the problems of selecting those applicants who will be accepted on to the courses. Despite the time, effort, and money that many schools invest in their selection processes, few have staff who are properly trained in selection theory and techniques, and in

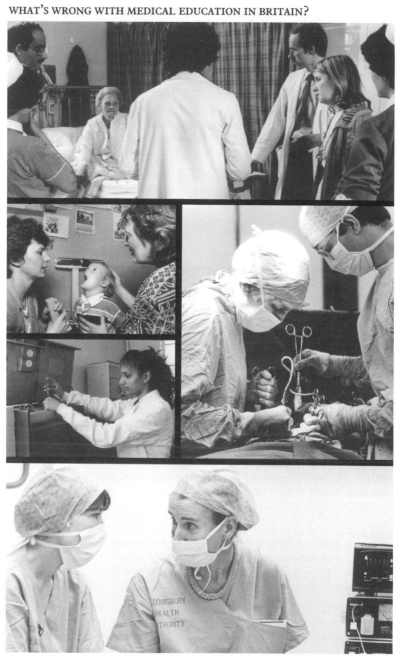

Doctors are now expected to work in multidisciplinary teams, not automatically as their leaders

4

many cases the processes are amateurish and depend more on luck than design for their success. This does not, however, mean that schools should spend a lot of effort in training staff to select students. Given the huge range of career options open to newly qualified doctors and the fact that all specialties in Britain now have formal postgraduate training schemes, it may be a waste of time to agonise too much about the type of student who should be allowed to enter the course. In view of the small pool of applicants available it seems unlikely that changing the selection process will have a major impact on the end product. I shall explore this dilemma in more detail in the next chapter.

What and how should we teach?

Perhaps the most difficult problem facing medical education is deciding how the course should be adapted to meet changing needs. The GMC and the King's Fund inquiry have identified curriculum overload as a major problem. Medical facts go out of date so quickly and medical information expands so fast that the most important skill for medical students to acquire is probably the ability to identify gaps in their knowledge and go about finding out for themselves the answers to the problems they face. Only then can they hope to be able to keep up with the changes that will occur during their professional lives.

The GMC has called for the introduction of a "core curriculum" taking up about two thirds of the total curriculum time, with the remainder available for students to pursue their own interests and study "options" in depth (box, p 8).[1] This leaves the medical schools with the huge problems of defining the core that all students must study and introducing facilities to encourage them to make good use of their private study time. A plethora of techniques for implementing such changes has grown up, and terms like "problem based," "self directed," and "student centred" abound in discussions about curriculum reform. Do these strategies really hold the key to successful changes in undergraduate teaching, and is the use of such jargon essential to clear discussion of the possible solutions or merely an elitist muddying of the waters that effectively excludes the doctors who do most of the teaching from contributing to the debates? Later I shall look at some of the suggested aims and strategies for reform of medical curricula. In particular, I shall discuss the SPICES model proposed by Professor Ron Harden of the Centre for Medical

Education at the University of Dundee, which is a valuable tool in weighing the pros and cons of some of the currently fashionable techniques.[8]

If schools do decide to adopt new teaching strategies do they have the staff to implement them? Experts in medical education, like Ron Harden, emphasise the need for staff development to ensure that such changes are properly implemented. A recent review on behalf of the Committee of Vice Chancellors and Principals of the Universities of the United Kingdom called for "training and development opportunities [to be] available to all staff who wish to prepare themselves for teaching excellence,"[9] and the King's Fund inquiry stated that "staff development programmes are needed not only to make teaching a more professional activity, but to help in developing a shared view of the philosophy of the medical school and to ensure that all staff work together to help students achieve the objectives of the course."[2] No effective changes can be expected in medical education unless staff are given the resources to implement the theories. Achieving this is another major problem facing our present system, and in subsequent articles I shall describe some of the attempts that have been made to give teaching the recognition it deserves.

Whose problems are they?

The GMC has statutory responsibility for medical education in Britain, but the day to day organisation is left largely to the individual schools. The education committee of the GMC issues regular recommendations to guide the schools and coordinates a system of regular visits to ensure that standards are maintained. In theory the GMC can refuse to recognise the qualifications of a particular school for the purposes of provisional registration of its graduates. In practice, however, these powers are not exercised — mainly because the council has no real option for disciplinary procedures short of derecognition of a whole course — with the devastating implications for the students in training. Thus, although the education committee can make recommendations, it can do little to enforce them. This is one of the greatest problems with our system of medical education, and the latest consultation document issued by the GMC hints at its frustration at the failure of the schools to implement the educational reforms proposed by the council in 1980, when it called for a reduction in the factual overload in the curriculum and the promotion of self education and critical thought.[1]

Medical schools are funded mainly by the Department for Education and Science through the Universities Funding Council. The funding of the clinical part of the medical course has always relied on a large measure of good will, with NHS staff teaching medical students and university staff providing services for NHS patients on a "knock for knock" basis. The NHS provides additional funds—the service increment for teaching and research, SIFTR ("ACTR" in Scotland, "STAR" in Northern Ireland)—to help offset the additional costs to hospitals of providing facilities for medical education. The recent reforms of the NHS and the need for tighter financial accounting led to worries that there would be great problems in identifying and allocating SIFTR funds and loss of the traditional good will between the universities and the NHS.[10 11] In practice the impact of the reforms has not been as great as had been feared,[12] and in some ways the emergence of a market economy may empower medical schools to demand the quality of medical education they require.

The cumbersome organisation of our medical education system, with responsibility for quality resting with the GMC and for funding shared between the education and health departments, means that no single body is in a position to supervise changes. We are already at a stage where many of the problems have been identified and some solutions have been suggested, but can we actually move forwards and implement effective change?

Time ripe for change

Many people are trying to find solutions to the problems in medical education, but perhaps the two clearest leads in recent years have come from the GMC and the King's Fund.[1 2] Both emphasise the need to reduce the factual load in the medical curriculum and encourage students to develop their skills at directing their own learning in preparation for continued education beyond university. The emphasis has shifted from absorbing medical facts to acquiring the knowledge, skills, and attitudes thought to be desirable in a modern doctor. The importance of postgraduate learning is emphasised, with basic medical education seen as only part of a continuum. The need for training in manipulating information technology to assist continued learning is recognised.

There is actually very little new in these ideas. By the end of the nineteenth century the GMC had recognised the problem of

---

GMC recommendations on undergraduate medical education

● Reduce excessive burden of factual information in the course—probably by dedicating two thirds of the course to a common "core" and allowing students to spend one third of their time on a series of "options," in which they could study selected subjects in more depth

● Introduce a substantial component of problem based learning

● Provide early clinical contact

● Ensure that all students develop a firm understanding of the scientific method

---

curriculum overload. In 1957 the GMC expressed concern about students tending to "concentrate their attention unduly on memorising factual data" and stated that the primary task of the medical course was "to instruct less and to educate more."[13] The latest consultation document issued by the GMC is largely the result of the education committee's disappointment at the failure of medical schools to respond to recommendations issued in 1980.[14] The philosophy underpinning the desirability of change has not altered substantially for decades—so why has nothing happened, and can it now?

Change on any great scale is disruptive and can be expensive. Medicine is a conservative profession, with high regard for old institutions and a tendency to assume that a system that worked well in the past should be preserved. But new forces are now driving change in medicine in general and medical education in particular.

The role of doctors has changed out of all recognition in recent decades. All are now expected to undertake higher specialist training and to work in multidisciplinary teams. Some of their traditional tasks are now done by other professionals. Changing work patterns for groups like nurses, pharmacists, social workers, and paramedical technicians have altered the role of doctors and in many cases replaced it. Doctors are no longer the automatic team leaders. Many members of the public do not remember life before the NHS and there is no longer an unquestioning gratitude and acceptance of what the doctor says and does. The public is increasingly well informed about medical matters and aware of its role in funding health care. The medical profession is having to be more accountable for the way in which it spends taxpayers' money.

Doctors have changed too. Increasingly they are demanding the right to have lives outside their jobs. It is no longer unthinkable to want a family life as well as a career.[5] Evidence is slowly emerging that those doctors who are most well rounded as individuals may also be the best at empathising and communicating with patients, leading to suggestions that "survival of the fittest" may not be survival of the best.[3] High salaries and prestige have been whittled away and no longer compensate for poor working conditions. It is becoming harder to "sell" medicine as a career option to school leavers, and this is reflected in reduced numbers of people applying for places in medical school.[15]

Changes in the provision of medical services are also having profound effects.[16] Technological developments allow rapid, minimally invasive investigations and treatments; cost implications discourage long inpatient stays; and growing emphasis on health promotion and disease prevention is shifting health care into the community.

All of these factors are affecting the way in which medicine is taught. The traditional teaching hospitals are no longer the only or best places to train doctors for the twenty first century. Change is inevitable and is currently being driven by pressures other than educational theory. If we can use the opportunity to direct some of the changes in line with desired educational principles we may achieve more in the next decade than we have done in the past century.

1 General Medical Council. *Undergraduate medical education.* London: GMC, 1991. (Discussion document by working party of GMC education committee.)
2 Towle A. *Critical thinking. The future of undergraduate medical education.* London: King's Fund Centre, 1991.
3 Firth-Cozens J. Stress in medical undergraduates and house officers. *Br J Hosp Med* 1989;**41**:161-4.
4 Firth-Cozens J. Emotional distress in junior house officers. *BMJ* 1987;**295**: 533-5.
5 Allen I. *Any room at the top? A study of doctors and their careers.* London: Policy Studies Institute, 1988.
6 Dillner L. The road to disenchantment. *BMJ* 1992;**305**:1103.
7 British Medical Association. *Stress and the medical profession.* London: BMA, 1992.
8 Harden RM, Sowden S, Dunn WR. Some educational strategies in curriculum development: the SPICES model. *Med Educ* 1984;**18**:284-97.
9 Elton L, Partington P. *Teaching standards and excellence in higher education. Developing a culture for quality.* Sheffield: Committee of Vice Chancellors and Principals of the Universities of the United Kingdom, 1992.
10 Secretaries of State for Health, Wales, Northern Ireland, and Scotland. *Working for patients.* London: HMSO, 1989. (Cm 555.)
11 Universities Funding Council Medical Committee. *First report on the effects of the NHS reforms on medical and dental education and research.* London: UFC, 1991.
12 Universities Funding Council Medical Committee. *Second report on the effects of the NHS reforms on medical and dental education and research.* London: UFC, 1992.

13 General Medical Council. *Recommendations as to the medical curriculum.* London: GMC, 1957.
14 General Medical Council. *Recommendations on basic medical education.* London: GMC Education Committee, 1980.
15 McManus C, Lockwood D. Medical education, training and research. In: Beck E, Lonsdale S, Newman S, Patterson D, eds. *In the best of health? The status and future of health care in the UK.* London: Chapman and Hall, 1992.
16 Stocking B. *Medical advances. The future shape of acute services.* London: King's Fund, 1992.

Selecting students

Medicine is often seen as a difficult university subject to enter, with medical schools choosing only the cream of students from many eager applicants. Certainly many schools spend considerable time, effort, and money on their selection process, but are they really getting a good return on this investment? Do we get the sort of medical students and doctors that we want? Are we even clear about what we want? Does it matter, anyway?

What do we want?

If medicine was simply a degree course like any other there would be little need for elaborate selection processes. Minimum scholastic achievement could be defined before entry to ensure that students had a fair chance of keeping up with the course, but places could then be awarded by lottery.

Most people, however, see the medical course as a vocational training. Applicants are expected to make medicine their career. Candidates are asked "Why do you want to be a doctor?" not "Why do you want to study medicine?" This is in sharp contrast with other degree courses. We do not, for example, expect all graduates in English to write or teach for a living. Nor do we insist that graduates from other facilities should "repay" society by obtaining any employment, much less in a specified field. A spattering of students who study medicine for its own sake might even enhance the educational climate in many of our medical schools.

If we assume, however, that medical education will continue, for

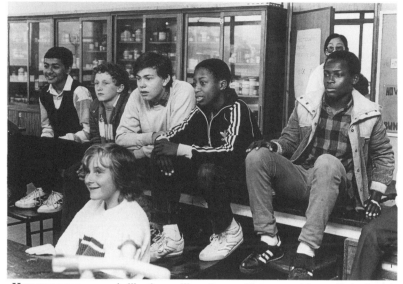

How many young people like these will apply to and be accepted by medical schools?

now, to be about training doctors then the selection process becomes one of choosing people who will make good doctors. This immediately raises the problem of defining a good doctor. Is there really an essential common core of knowledge, skills, and attitudes that all doctors should have? In a profession like medicine there may well be niches for all—whatever their particular interests, skills, and weaknesses. Specific aptitudes are doubtless important in selecting people for specialist training, but their relevance at the undergraduate stage is much less obvious.

Is there an end product?

If we could clearly identify the aims of undergraduate medical education we could begin to decide how best to select medical students. The General Medical Council defines the principal objective of basic medical education as providing "the knowledge, skills and attitudes which will provide a firm basis for future vocational training."[1]

The only immediate requirement is to produce a graduate who can function as a preregistration house officer. This should enable an essential core of factual knowledge and clinical skills to be defined that all doctors should have mastered by the end of the course. They will then have to embark on a protracted postgraduate education in their chosen specialty. All medical graduates should therefore have the skills to enable them to continue learning beyond university.

In recent years the trend has been for medical schools to select only the most academically gifted applicants, with standard offers of places often depending on acquiring three "A" grades at A level. This attitude is now changing, more schools acknowledging that people with only moderate academic achievement can cope well with the course and often have more to offer in terms of personal skills, attitudes, and experience. Dr John Foreman, subdean of University College and Middlesex School of Medicine, University College, London, recently explained the school's reasons for setting low minimum requirements for entry: "Our standard offer of C, C, C is the lowest in the country. . . . We strongly believe C, C, C reflects the level of academic ability needed to follow the course. It gives us the scope to admit people below the academic average for medicine, but who possess other qualities we deem to be more important."[2] Schools like Newcastle (box) and University College and Middlesex School of Medicine now place more emphasis on personality and

---

Student selection at the medical school, University of Newcastle upon Tyne

- All UCCA forms are screened to ensure minimum scholastic achievement on the basis of GCSE results and predicted A level grades
- Above threshold level, scholastic achievement plays no further part in the selection process
- All students achieving the threshold for scholastic achievement are graded 1 to 5 on other aspects of their applications. Attention is paid to excellence outside academic life, community service, social activities, etc
- All applicants scoring 5 and some of those scoring 4 are invited for interview
- During interview academic ability is taken for granted
- Attention is again directed to other aspects of the candidate's personality and interests
- Awareness of special features of the Newcastle curriculum and evidence of genuine interest in innovative curricula (based on other courses listed on UCCA form) carry considerable weight

---

motivation in selecting students and have low minimum requirements for A level grades at entry (although in practice most of their entrants obtain grades well above the required minimum).

Some schools select students whom they believe are particularly suited to the specific course on offer. McMaster University in Canada has an unusual medical course based almost entirely on self directed learning in small tutorial groups. There are no formal examinations, and students are expected to take on much of the responsibility for what they learn. McMaster has broad entry criteria, taking students who have much lower academic achievements than the norm for North American medical courses. The students also tend to be older than those in other schools. They are, however, carefully selected on the basis of their skills at directing their own learning and working in small groups (box).[3] Although many of the entrants would have failed to obtain a place in other North American medical schools, they seem to cope as well as other students during the course and beyond.[4-6]

What should we look for?

We now accept that no doctor can learn all that there is to know about medicine and that medical facts go out of date quickly. The ability to identify gaps in one's own knowledge, seek out new information, assess it sensibly, and act on the new knowledge is more important than the ability to absorb vast amounts of factual informa-

---

Student selection at McMaster University, Hamilton, Ontario, Canada

Students are selected at McMaster on the basis of their performance during a simulated tutorial designed to test their skills at problem solving in small groups. The aim is to select students in a way that reflects the pattern of study in the school.[3]

• Applicants are allocated to tutorial groups of five or six, with a tutor for each group

• Each tutorial lasts about 45 minutes, during which the group tackles two unstructured problems

• About half way through the tutorial candidates are asked to summarise how well they think they are functioning in the group

• A team of assessors observes the tutorial through one way mirror and assesses how well each candidate performs within the group

---

tion and perform well in tests of recall. Dr Chris McManus, from St Mary's Hospital, Paddington, who has conducted extensive research into how medical students learn, believes that learning styles are better predictors of university performance than are A level results. Certainly among medical students poor performance in examinations is hardly ever the result of low academic ability.[7]

Ideally we should be selecting medical students who have the attitudes and learning styles that will help them to continue lifelong education. Three main types of learning style have been identified.[8] A shallow learner adopts rote learning and may perform well in tests of short term recall, but this style does not correlate well with deep understanding of a problem. A deep learner grasps the underlying concepts and understands the problem rather than memorising the facts. A strategic learner uses features of both styles and adapts as required by the specific task. A deep learner will be better able than a shallow learner to cope with the ongoing demands of a subject like medicine. A strategic learner may also cope well.

Chris McManus has found that people can readily adopt shallow learning techniques, but that deep learning skills are much harder to acquire. In one study the students who performed badly in end of term examinations quickly adopted shallow techniques in response to the pressures of the next exam. This led rapidly to a downward spiral of achievement.[7] Chris McManus thinks that an important response to this problem is to modify the examination format to reduce factual recall and encourage understanding of the underlying principles, but he also thinks that we should try to select students who have an established deep learning style. Admissions tutors might do better to select on the basis of psychometric testing rather than GCSE and A level grades.

Essentials of the selection process

Despite the time and money that many schools spend on their selection procedures the methods are, on the whole, amateurish and haphazard. Most schools rely on the good will of a few motivated members of staff to assist the dean in sorting out applications. Many schools select entirely on the basis of information provided on the UCCA form. But even those that consider interviews to be important in identifying the traits most desirable in a medical student or doctor rarely train their staff in interviewing techniques. The small pool of volunteers for this difficult and time consuming task may allow some

15

consistency of approach within each school, but it is no guarantee of excellence.

Dr Brian Jolly of St Bartholomew's Hospital Medical School, London (which has a written protocol to guide selectors), agrees that the system in many schools is haphazard but questions whether it would really be cost effective to undertake extensive training of those taking part. He thinks that there are so many and varied opportunities after graduation in medicine that selectors should not agonise too much about choosing the "right sort" of undergraduate.

There is, however, one essential feature of selection processes that all schools should monitor and enforce — the system must be fair.[9] In 1987 the preliminary screening programme at St George's Hospital Medical School was discovered to be discriminating against female applicants and those with non-European sounding surnames.[10-12] The problem was identified only because the preliminary screening was being computerised, and similar covert discrimination was undoubtedly common in other schools. The resulting outcry led to the introduction of ethnic monitoring of applicants and entrants to medical schools.[13] This ensures that racial discrimination does not happen once people have applied for medical school, but a more difficult problem is ensuring that there is no discrimination by default, with people from ethnic minorities failing to apply at all. Across Britain, students from Asian backgrounds are now overrepresented in proportion to their numbers in the community, and Chris McManus thinks that this reflects a general trend for Asian families to encourage their children to obtain portable professional qualifications. There is still, however, a dearth of applicants to British medical schools from African and Caribbean backgrounds and no sign of attempts to tackle the problem.

Nor is race the only area for possible discrimination. We may now have almost equal numbers of male and female medical students in Britain, but we have been less successful in ensuring a mix of social class backgrounds. The social class mix of British medical students has changed little in the past 30 years, and the latest figures available from UCCA confirm that 31% of applicants and 38% of acceptances in 1991 came from professional families (the corresponding figures for skilled manual workers and unskilled workers being 8% and 7% and 0·7% and 0·4% respectively). Recent trends like the student loan scheme and the recession will further discourage applicants from poorer backgrounds.

Another area of potential discrimination is the age of the applicant.

Despite the fact that mature students cope well with the medical course and are often thought to have a stabilising influence on the younger students, most medical schools actively discriminate against the oldest applicants—usually on the basis of the length of the postgraduate training for doctors. Universities have no real justification for basing decisions on an applicant's hypothesised subsequent career, and Chris McManus suggests that in some countries with better established antidiscrimination laws, such as the United States, the legality of such an approach could be challenged effectively through the courts.

The rationing myth

Most medical schools assume that their selection process serves an important rationing function, ensuring that only the best of the vast number of eager applicants gain places. Although individual schools may receive 10 or more applications for each place, the number of people applying to study medicine is falling despite an overall trend for more people to enter tertiary education. UCCA data confirm that applications for places at British medical schools fell by 2·7% between 1985 and 1991, while the total number of applicants for all university places rose by 29·8%. Although no formal studies have investigated the reasons, many people I have spoken to suggest that the public image of medicine as a career has taken a severe knocking in recent years with publicity about the long hours of work, a fall in doctors' salaries relative to other professions, and studies showing high levels of dissatisfaction among medical students and young doctors.[14-16]

Once allowance is made for the multiple applications permitted on the UCCA form there are actually only two applicants for each place on a medical course in British universities. The selection process is becoming as much a case of students choosing schools as schools selecting students. Dr Reg Jordan, the academic subdean at Newcastle, recognises this. "We want to offer places to students who really want to be here." He sees that as particularly important, given that Newcastle has an unusual course with considerable integration between the basic and clinical sciences and large elements of self directed learning. If as a result of recent moves by the GMC[17] schools become more diverse in the content and style of their courses this element of students choosing schools may become even more pronounced.

17

Improving selection

Despite the time and money invested in selecting students for medical schools the systems are unlikely to identify those most suited to recent changes in medicine. More effort should be directed to selecting for desired learning styles and less emphasis placed on academic success at school. Any system must be fair, and in particular we need to find ways of encouraging applicants from all social classes and ethnic groups. Given the small and dwindling pool of applicants to medical schools, we should be realistic about how influential the selection process can be in shaping the final product. If this is to change we must encourage more applicants by reversing recent negative images of medicine as a career.

1 General Medical Council. *Recommendations on basic medical education.* London: GMC, 1980.
2 Wade G. Diagnosing the doctors. *The Guardian* 1991 Nov 6: 23.
3 Mitchell DLM, Pallie W, McAuley RG. The simulated tutorial. *British Journal of Medical Education* 1975;**9**:133-9.
4 Woodward CA. The effects of the innovations in medical education at McMaster: a report on follow-up studies. *MEDUCS* 1989;**2**:64-8.
5 Woodward CA, Ferrier BM. Perspectives of graduates two or five years after graduation from a three year medical school. *Journal of Medical Education* 1982;**57**:294-302.
6 Ferrier BM, Woodward CA. Does premedical academic background influence medical graduates' perceptions of their medical school or their subsequent career paths and decisions? *Med Educ* 1983;**17**:72-8.
7 Tooth D, Tonge K, McManus IC. Anxiety and study methods in preclinical students: causal relation to examination performance. *Med Educ* 1989;**23**: 416-21.
8 Newble DI, Entwistle NJ. Learning styles and approaches: implications for medical education. *Med Educ* 1986;**20**:162-75.
9 Powis DA, McManus IC, Cleave-Hogg D. Selection of medical students: philosophic, political, social, and educational bases. *Teaching and Learning in Medicine* 1992;**4**:25-34.
10 Commission for Racial Equality. *Medical school admissions: report of a formal investigation into St George's Hospital Medical School.* London: CRE, 1988.
11 Lowry S, Macpherson G. A blot on the profession. *BMJ* 1988;**296**:657-8.
12 McManus IC, Richards P, Maitlis SL. Prospective study of the disadvantage of people from ethnic minority groups applying to medical schools in the United Kingdom. *BMJ* 1989;**298**:723-6.
13 McManus IC, Maitlis SL, Richards P. Identifying medical school applicants from ethnic minorities. *Studies in Higher Education* 1990;**15**:57-73.
14 Allen I. *Doctors and their careers.* London: Policy Studies Institute, 1988.
15 Firth-Cozens J. Emotional distress in junior house officers. *BMJ* 1987;**295**: 533-6.
16 Firth-Cozens J. Stress in medical undergraduates and house officers. *Br J Hosp Med* 1989;**41**:161-4.
17 General Medical Council. *Undergraduate medical education: a consultation document.* London: GMC, 1991.

Curriculum design

In 1991 the General Medical Council expressed concern at the response of many students to the present course—"it is distressing to see the progressive disenchantment of many of them as they work their way through the course. Imagination and curiosity are soon dulled."[1] It also highlighted the overburdened curriculum, with undue emphasis on the passive acquisition of facts that were soon forgotten, as a major area for reform. Instead, the council wants more promotion of self directed learning skills and cultivation of the attitudes needed to keep up to date with a rapidly changing subject like medicine.

The council defined the primary aim of the undergraduate course in terms of acquiring "an understanding of health and disease, and of the prevention and management of the latter, in the context of the whole individual in his or her place in the family and society." To this end it set out some essential components of the course (box).

It defined the second aim of the course as developing "an attitude to learning that is based on curiosity and the exploration of knowledge" and stated its intention to "reduce the excessive burden of information in the existing undergraduate course." The council recommends that schools should substantially reduce the amount of face to face teaching that goes on and instead offer support and guidance for students to direct their own learning. Other recommendations include a clinical component from day 1 and the need to acquire an understanding of scientific method.

The most striking feature of the new proposals is the introduction of the concept of a "core" curriculum and "options." The core, which

Features that GMC considers to be essential aspects of the undergraduate curriculum

- Knowledge and understanding of the scientific basis of medicine
- Introduction to a range of problems presenting to doctors and a range of possible solutions
- Understanding of basic disease processes
- Ability to elicit history and perform physical examination
- Understanding of mental illness and psychological responses to physical illness
- Appreciation of health promotion and disease prevention
- Understanding of principles of therapy and disease management
- Understanding of reproductive cycle
- Understanding of human relationships
- Understanding of organisation of health services
- Awareness of ethical and legal responsibilities of doctors
- Skill in essential clinical procedures like cardiopulmonary resuscitation
- Development of the capacity for self audit

might vary slightly from school to school, would be required of all students, but the optional aspects would allow in depth study of some aspects which the students would largely select for themselves. Professor David Shaw, chairman of the GMC's education committee, now admits that the choice of the word "options" was unfortunate, as a major stumbling block in negotiations about the proposals has been the unwillingness of staff to admit that their subject does not have to be part of the core. Despite the semantic problems, however, the council is convinced that the educational objectives of the under-graduate curriculum can best be achieved by reducing the compulsory elements to not more than two thirds of the total course time. In fact, it is unlikely that the options would be a dumping ground for minor specialties. More probably they would develop as an opportunity for project work or electives, giving a deeper exploration of parts of the core curriculum that had particularly interested the student.

Because the council recognised that the proposed changes will mean considerable upheaval for many schools it decided to issue a consultation document outlining its proposals. It accepted that full implementation would probably take 10 years. The council has now received responses from the medical schools and other interested bodies and is deciding on the next step.

National consensus

The GMC is not the only organisation looking at the current problems in British medical education. In 1990 the King's Fund Centre, in collaboration with St Bartholomew's Medical School and City and Hackney Health Authority, London, set up a national inquiry into the subject, with the aim of establishing guidelines for redesigning the undergraduate curriculum. The inquiry used a modified Delphi technique to reach consensus through several rounds of consultation. In the first round participants were sent a series of propositions and questions on medical education and asked to suggest other topics that should be covered. In the second round a new list was circulated and participants asked to comment on that. In round 3 a summary of the comments received after round 2 was circulated for additional comments and to allow participants to see the extent of consensus emerging. The consultation ended with a conference in April 1991, from which written recommendations were issued.[2] The inquiry confirmed that there is widespread agreement among medical teachers that the undergraduate course is overcrowded and inhibits students from critical and creative thinking. The key issues identified by the inquiry are summarised in the box.

Key issues in curriculum development identified by the King's Fund inquiry

● Need to define core knowledge, skills, and attitudes in line with the GMC's recommendations—possibly by setting up a national advisory group
● Integration of preclinical and clinical teaching by redesigning the curriculum as a continuum
● Introduction of self directed learning
● Development of new methods of student assessment to test all desired knowledge, skills, and attitudes
● Proper recognition for medical teachers, with teaching commitments specified in contracts, audit of teaching quality, and appropriate financial rewards for teaching excellence
● Staff development to allow teachers to take on their new roles
● More teaching in outpatient clinics, general practice and community settings, and skills laboratories
● Proper management of change within medical schools, with appropriate funding and evaluation of the process

---

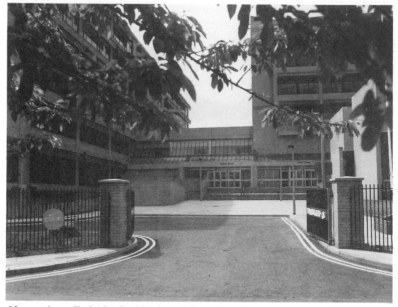

Newcastle medical school, which has engineered a series of major innovative changes in its curriculum since 1962

Many of the identified aims of an ideal curriculum are in line with the GMC's recommendations, but the inquiry also looked at barriers to implementing change and how they might be overcome. Among factors likely to aid change the report identified the strong lead from the GMC, the introduction of university contracts and NHS job plans giving deans the opportunity to specify teaching commitments, and the opportunity to use the allocation of SIFTR money to add weight to these demands. The low status of teachers in medical education, the departmental organisation of many courses, and the traditional divide between the basic sciences and the clinical course were identified as major barriers to change.

The report also emphasised that many medical schools were already some way along the road to implementing desired change but that the absence of a national forum for the exchange of ideas and information meant that time was being wasted by individual units reinventing the wheel and failing to learn from other people's mistakes. Perhaps the most useful thing to come out of the King's Fund initiative has been the establishment of a national forum for the exchange of information about medical education initiatives (box).

Unhappy staff, unhappy students?

St Bartholomew's Hospital Medical School was closely concerned with the King's Fund in setting up its inquiry into medical education, and it is one of the schools that has already made progress in implementing changes in line with the GMC's proposals. The driving force behind these changes has been the dean, Lesley Rees, who was horrified at the transformation of eager, bright school leavers into dull, demoralised doctors in five short years. She organised a series of surveys of students and recent graduates and confirmed that they thought the course was overcrowded and relied too heavily on the passive recall of facts and that the preclinical course had too little obvious clinical relevance. A survey of the teachers in the preclinical departments found that they too were unhappy. They were bored by what they had to teach and demoralised by the effects of the course on their pupils.

A curriculum steering group was convened. All the members had an interest in medical education, but no attempt was made to ensure that all departments were represented. The school has now introduced an innovative preclinical course, although the clinical years have yet to be tackled. Within the new course there is considerable integration of subjects, so that departmental boundaries are blurred, lectures are limited to a maximum of two a day, and there is a large element of community based education and teaching of communication skills. The first group of students to follow the new course did well, Brian Jolly told me, but the examination results for the second year were disappointing. The school is trying to identify why this happened, but preliminary comments from the students suggest that they were not all fully prepared for the responsibility of self directed learning — "Initially we didn't know how to begin and wasted

---

"Change in Medical Education"

"Change in Medical Education" is a network of people interested in sharing information and ideas about the current problems and changes in medical education. It was set up by the King's Fund after publication of its inquiry into these issues, and members receive a quarterly newsletter and invitations to conferences, workshops, and seminars. Anyone interested in joining should contact Dr Angela Towle at the King's Fund Centre, 126 Albert Street, London NW1 7NF.

many hours wondering where to find information." There is no point in introducing change unless all those concerned understand the processes.

Change as a dynamic process

Innovative attitudes to medical education are not new, even in Britain. Newcastle medical school (fig 1) has undergone a series of major innovative changes starting in 1962. Throughout, the aim has been to break down the traditional barriers between clinical and preclinical studies by teaching around the major systems of the body rather than along traditional departmental lines.[3] The course has undergone three major revisions—in 1962, 1976, and 1988. The present course consists of modules of teaching based on the major organ systems. Each module is controlled by an interdisciplinary system course subcommittee of students and staff from the basic and clinical sciences, which reports eventually to the faculty teaching committee chaired by the dean.

Reg Jordan emphasises that effective curriculum development is an ongoing process: "Change is an ongoing dynamic process, with peaks and troughs." The subcommittees at Newcastle are constantly monitoring and refining the courses that they supervise, but on top of that there have been three major revisions of the overall policy. The first two were primarily concerned with integrating the basic sciences and clinical teaching. By the mid-1980s, however, it was apparent that the course was still overloaded, and the teaching committee was also concerned that students were not developing their self learning potential properly. The committee examined the factual content of the first year of the course and succeeded in redefining the core of factual information to be included. The formal, timetabled element of the course was thus reduced by a quarter, and about half of the total teaching time in the week is now available for private study. Reg Jordan thinks that as well as defining core knowledge clearly schools have a duty to "make a clear statement about what students do not need to learn" as this helps to reduce student anxiety in courses with a large element of self directed learning.

During the most recent reorganisation of the Newcastle curriculum the teaching committee also introduced a new system of student assessment in the hope of shifting the emphasis from rote learning of facts to the development of learning skills and deeper understanding of underlying principles. More emphasis is now placed on "open

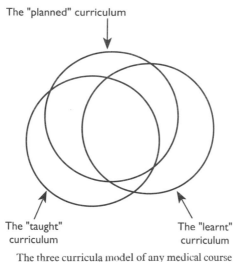

The "planned" curriculum

The "taught" curriculum

The "learnt" curriculum

The three curricula model of any medical course

hook" in couise assessments by means of essays, longer dissertations, and practical projects. These are supplemented by more traditional multiple choice question papers, data interpretation and objective structured practical examinations, short answer papers, and essays.

The first group of students to complete the new course graduated in 1992, so formal evaluation of the success of the approach is still limited. So far, however, feedback from the students has been encouraging, although some members of staff are still worried that there has been "change for change's sake." Reg Jordan emphasises that it is often impossible to prove that a particular way of teaching is "better" than any other but that it "feels more sensible to teach this way."

The developments at St Bartholomew's and Newcastle prove that if a few key members of staff are willing to make a stand the required factual content of the undergraduate medical course can be defined and reduced. This is encouraging, given the caution expressed by some respondents to the King's Fund inquiry.[2] Nevertheless, it may still be more effective to set up a national advisory panel to define the core required of all students, as suggested in the King's Fund report, than to leave the brave to introduce change and the cautious to do nothing.

The three curricula model

It is not enough merely to define the teaching content of a course. What teachers teach and what students learn may not be the same. Dr Colin Coles, an educational psychologist from Southampton, suggests that the education process can be illustrated by a three curricula model (figure). One curriculum is that which the faculty intends should be taught (the "planned" curriculum); another consists of what the teachers do, in fact, teach (the "taught" curriculum); and the third is what the students actually learn (the "learnt" curriculum). The degree of overlap among these curricula will vary, and any attempt to change a course needs to take account of all three aspects. Concentrating solely on what you plan to teach may have little impact on what students learn.

1 General Medical Council. *Undergraduate medical education. The need for change.* London: GMC, 1991.
2 Towle A. *Critical thinking: the future of undergraduate medical education.* London: King's Fund Centre, 1991.
3 Walton JN. On training tomorrow's doctors: the Newcastle curriculum revised and reconstructed. *BMJ* 1977;i:1262-5.

Strategies for implementing curriculum change

What strategies can be used to implement the desired reforms proposed by the General Medical Council?[1] Most people accept that the way in which a subject is taught can have as much impact on what students learn as the content of the course. A recent review by the Oxford Centre for Staff Development identified five aspects of educational programmes that are associated with students adopting undesirable shallow learning techniques and failing to grasp the underlying principles of the topic.[2] The five features are heavy workload; excessive amount of course material; little opportunity to pursue subjects in depth; little choice over topics or methods of study; and an anxiety provoking assessment system that rewards or tolerates regurgitation of factual information.

Reg Jordan likes to quote these points when talking about medical education because people inevitably assume that they are describing the traditional British medical course. In fact, none of the studies on which they are based was of medical education, although there is no reason why the general principles should not apply more widely. Many of the strategies that have been used to implement change in medical curricula are designed to tackle such problems with the traditional course.

Much discussion about curriculum strategy is couched in educational jargon that may exclude many people from debates about the best approach. There is also a danger that people will become obsessed with the processes and forget the underlying aims. This danger has been highlighted by Professor Ron Harden and his colleagues at the Centre for Medical Education at the University of

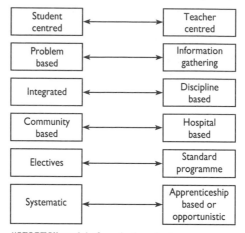

"SPICES" model of curriculum design

Dundee. They warn that too often the strategic concepts become "a thin gold veneer to a curriculum package" or come to be "ends in themselves, while the real aims and purposes of the curriculum are forgotten." In an attempt to encourage schools to think about why they are adopting certain approaches the centre has developed a model for curriculum design based on six key strategic concepts.[3] The "SPICES" model represents the innovative extremes of six spectra (figure), and staff should consider the pros and cons of each extreme before deciding what approach works best in their setting. I shall use the SPICES model to look at some common strategic approaches to change in medical education.

Student centred learning

Many traditional medical courses are essentially teacher centred, with staff defining the objectives for the course, the course content, the learning resources and teaching methods to be used, and the pace of teaching and methods of assessment. In a student centred system, however, the students take on much of the responsibility for these tasks. At its most extreme a student based course may follow the lines of the medical course at McMaster University in Canada. There the students learn in small groups with a member of staff available to advise if required but taking no part in selecting what or how they learn. The students are given a choice of clinical problems to tackle, and it is up to them to decide which aspects to pursue. They are responsible for defining the objectives of each new topic and choosing what resources to use in studying it. They may, for example, decide to work in the library or resources centre, or they may call in a clinical expert to give a tutorial to the group.

Less extreme approaches to shifting the focus on to students and away from teachers include simple changes like ensuring that formal teaching occurs at times and in settings that are convenient for the students, rather than being designed solely to fit in with staff commitments. This is especially important in postgraduate medical education, when students are under considerable pressure from the service aspects of their jobs. People do not learn well when they are tired or risk being interrupted to attend to other matters, and ensuring that teaching is geared to fit in with their other commitments makes it much easier for them to take full advantage of it. The Standing Committee on Postgraduate Medical Education has emphasised such potential benefits of a more student centred approach.[4]

Student centred learning is thought to increase motivation and enhance learning by shifting the emphasis from what is taught to what is actually learnt. It is also seen as a good preparation for continued learning beyond the confines of a formal course. There are disadvantages, however, and among these Professor Harden identifies the facts that student centred learning can be difficult to coordinate and administer; teacher centred approaches are often the most cost effective way of imparting a body of factual information to a large group of students; many teachers have not been trained in the special facilitating skills needed to assist in student centred learning; and unless students are familiar with how to direct their own learning they can be left floundering.

Problem based learning

In the past British medical schools have tended to concentrate on teaching facts which doctors then have to learn to marshal as required to tackle the problems that they face in clinical practice. The GMC has stated that we should move away from this approach and introduce a large element of "problem based learning" into the undergraduate curriculum.[1] The idea behind problem based learning is that students are presented with a real clinical situation and use it as a springboard from which to explore various topics. An elderly woman who falls and fractures her leg may, for example, form the basis for learning about

29

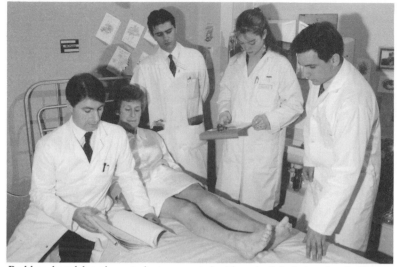

Problem based learning: students presented with real clinical situation facilitating exploration of other topics

the anatomy of the lower limb, the physiology of bone healing, the epidemiology of osteoporosis, the risks of immobilisation in the elderly, the pharmacology of acute pain relief, and the social consequences of disability. The hope is that this will feel more realistic than the traditional approach, so encouraging students to remain enthusiastic about what they are doing, and that it will be easier for them to recall what they have learnt because the service setting will be similar to the setting in which the facts were originally learnt.[5] Several new medical schools have based their courses almost entirely on problem based learning—the most well known being McMaster in Canada, Maastricht in the Netherlands, and Newcastle in Australia.

Problem based learning fits in well with integrated approaches, in which students study various aspects of a problem simultaneously (see below), and also works well in self directed learning programmes where the students choose which aspects of a problem to tackle. At McMaster, for example, the clinical problem outlined above might be presented to a tutorial group, but it would be up to the students themselves to identify the possible learning opportunities it presented and decide which of them to explore and in what detail. Because some of the most vocal advocates of problem based learning have been the new, innovative schools like McMaster there is a tendency for more traditional schools to assume that this is an approach that can be adopted only as part of a package including strategies like self directed learning, small group learning, or integrated learning. This is not necessarily so, and Dr Luis Branda, chairman of the programme for faculty development at McMaster, emphasises that elements of problem based learning can be incorporated into various types of curricula.[6] In fact, many doctors teaching in British hospitals use a problem based approach every day, although they may not think to call it that.

Relation with problem solving

A common difficulty when people talk about problem based learning is the assumption that it is the same as "problem solving." This is not so, and indeed if the aim was to solve clinical problems there would be limited applications of a problem based approach to teaching very inexperienced undergraduates. As people progress through medical training and acquire more knowledge and experience they may "solve" some of the problems that they encounter, but the aim of problem based learning is to provide a framework for teaching and learning, not to arrive at the correct solution.

Some exponents of problem based learning suggest that it is a good way of developing the problem solving skills that a doctor will need in clinical practice.[3] But there is little evidence that this is so. The development of clinical reasoning skills was studied in a random cross sectional sample of medical students from three years of the course at McMaster and a separate group of students from a single year, who were studied longitudinally throughout the course.[7] The students were observed in the clinical examination of a simulated patient, and their underlying reasoning processes were explored during subsequent review of the videotaped consultation.

Although the diagnostic and management skills of the students improved as they progressed through the course, there was little change in the processes they used to reach their conclusions. The authors concluded that despite the problem based approach to medical education at McMaster, the students did not develop problem solving skills. They simply acquired more knowledge, which allowed them to make more sensible hypotheses about what was going on.

This may, of course, be a reflection of the setting of the study. Students at McMaster are carefully selected for their skills at self directed learning and may be already good at problem solving.[8]

31

A problem based course might help students who do not already have well developed problem solving skills to acquire them. Colin Coles thinks that problem based learning encourages students to adopt desirable deep learning approaches (in which they acquire an understanding of the underlying principles of a problem rather than simply memorising superficial facts about it). He carried out a longitudinal study of students at two medical schools, one with a conventional curriculum and the other with a problem based approach. On entry the two groups had similar learning styles, but after only one year those in the conventional school showed a significant shift in their learning styles towards shallow techniques with emphasis on the rote learning of facts, while the students at the other school had maintained their desirable deep learning attitudes.[9]

Integrated courses

The traditional British medical course, as described in the first chapter, was clearly separated into preclinical and clinical sections.[10] Within each section topics were further divided by subject, discipline based departments taking on responsibility for teaching small, unconnected sections of the course. A recurrent criticism of this approach is that students fail to appreciate the relevance of what they learn in one part of the course to other aspects of the whole curriculum. Anecdotally this is widely recognised, most doctors admitting that they cannot remember much of what they learnt in the basic science courses at medical school. A survey of students and graduates at St Bartholomew's Hospital, London, confirmed that they thought much of the preclinical teaching was irrelevant, and the concept has also been accepted by organisations like the GMC and the King's Fund in their statements on the medical curriculum.[1 11]

Part of the problem is undoubtedly the overload of the medical course. Much of what is presented in preclinical courses is irrelevant to what a doctor really needs to know. Reg Jordan believes that curriculum designers should be brave enough to state clearly what students don't need to know, as well as what they should know. Chris McManus points out that most students who fail in medical courses do so in the preclinical years, when they are essentially studying courses and sitting exams that have been designed by non-medical staff. He questions whether these teachers should have such a large say in who does or does not become a doctor.

Some schools have gone a considerable way to reducing the content of the medical course, especially in the preclinical sciences. But there is still a problem that students also tend to forget the facts that are relevant to what comes later. Colin Coles emphasises that we tend to learn best when we learn in context. Facts are remembered most easily in a setting similar to the one in which they were learnt—a simple example being the difficulty we may have in putting a name to a familiar face met out of the usual setting. These notions have led increasingly to calls for the medical course to be integrated so that the traditional boundaries disappear and students see the relevance of what they are doing.

Horizontal and vertical integration

There are two major approaches to integrating medical courses, although the underlying concepts are similar. In horizontal integration the boundaries between parallel parts of the course are removed, and in vertical integration those between sequential areas are lost. The changes in St Bartholomew's preclinical course are a good example of horizontal integration, with loss of the traditional departmental responsibilities for sections of the course.[12]

The systems approach at Newcastle is another good example of integration—students learning the anatomy, physiology, and biochemistry of each major organ system together. The Newcastle course also illustrates the principle of vertical integration; here students learn the clinical aspects of the organ systems at the same time as they learn underlying science.[13]

Ron Harden's team in Dundee identifies several advantages of integrated teaching in medicine. For example, students are more motivated by seeing the relevance of what they are doing and more likely to remember what they learn because they are learning it in context. In addition, because they are learning about all aspects of a problem at the same time they are automatically adopting a holistic approach to clinical problems, which fits well with modern ideas about treating patients as whole people living in a community and not just as examples of particular disorders.[1] Integrated courses also encourage cooperation between staff from different departments and avoid wasteful duplication and repetition of effort by better coordination of the whole course.

There are some disadvantages, however. Unless great care is taken over coordinating the course, important topics may be overlooked. Reg Jordan believes that "the first step in integration is coordination," but this can be cumbersome and expensive, and discipline based teaching may simply be easier to set up.

Practical difficulties

There may also be practical restrictions on the amount of integration that is possible. At Newcastle it was fairly easy to provide vertical integration because the medical school has access to many hospital sites and a large number of willing clinical teachers. Brian Jolly points out, however, that at St Bartholomew's there is limited scope for vertical integration because the teaching site for the basic sciences course at Queen Mary College has access to only one hospital, at Mile End. Reg Jordan thinks that there is no single solution to the problems in medical education and emphasises that changes should take note of local contexts, including any historical and geographical considerations. Some schools may find it impossible to set up a fully integrated course from day 1 but might, for example, make use of a wedge structure in designing the curriculum so that both preclinical and clinical subjects are taught throughout the course, but with preclinical studies predominating in the early years and time devoted to clinical subjects increasing as the course progresses (figure).

Many teachers may find it hard to teach on an integrated course, and some of their enthusiasm may be lost if they do not feel that they are teaching their own subject. A preliminary assessment of the new horizontally integrated basic sciences course at St Bartholomew's has identified that staff find it difficult to set a truly integrated exam and that questions from various disciplines are juxtaposed rather than integrated.

Community based education

Recent changes in the provision of health services have led to increasing questions about whether traditional teaching hospitals are the best places to educate medical students. On 10 July 1992 the King's Fund Centre ran a conference which explored these ideas and examined the concept of community based education as a solution to many of them. Among the problems identified with our traditional hospital based system is that economic pressures and the opportunities created by modern technology mean that many patients now receive all of their treatment outside hospital or in day case units. Those who are admitted are often in hospital for a very short time and may not be available for teaching preclinical students about common

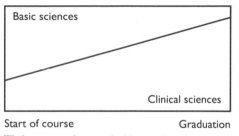

Wedge approach to vertical integration

conditions. Much of what goes on in hospitals now is so specialised as to be of limited use to undergraduate students anyway.

A possible solution is to move much of medical education into the community. Dr Nigel Oswald, from the department of general practice at Cambridge University, is a great advocate of this approach.[14 15] He emphasises that community based teaching is not about teaching general practice. It is a way of teaching general medicine in the community. In 1993 a group of four students at Cambridge started on a pilot project of 15 months of community based education in place of the traditional junior medical and surgical attachments and specialty rotations.

Seeing care in context

Among the perceived advantages of community based teaching is that students see patients in their own environments and get a clear understanding of how illness affects all aspects of a person's life. This is in line with recent calls from the GMC for undergraduates to study health and disease "in the context of the whole individual in his or her place in the family and society." Students also learn about how health services are provided, the importance of a team approach, and how primary and secondary services interact. They get a better idea of the relative importance of various conditions for the whole community and have more exposure to the health promotion and disease prevention aspects of medicine that the GMC wants emphasised in the undergraduate curriculum.[1]

There are, however, some advantages of a hospital based course. The organisation is much simpler—a major problem with community based teaching is that students must learn in small groups and there are numerous logistic problems in ensuring adequate accommodation, transport, and support services for them when they are widely

35

scattered from the school base. When the Cambridge scheme starts next year, for example, only students with their own cars will be able to volunteer, as others might not be able to visit patients at night, attend outpatient clinics, or follow patients to casualty departments as required. Students may actually resent the loss of a group identity when they are farmed out in small groups away from their medical schools. There may also be difficulty in recruiting enough suitable tutors to supervise students in the community, although Nigel Oswald points to the enthusiasm with which general practitioners have found places for postgraduate trainees as evidence that this can be overcome. Whether or not the system could cope with large numbers of undergraduate students remains to be seen, especially as they would need supervision and tutoring on a broader base than merely the general practice aspects of a case.

Electives

One of the most radical proposals in the latest consultation document issued by the education committee of the GMC is that we should move away from our traditional approach of all students studying the same course and introduce a system of a common "core" with "options."[1] The main aims behind this idea are the need to reduce the factual load in the curriculum and the desire to encourage students to develop skills in learning for themselves. The GMC now regrets the choice of the term "options," because of its connotation as something non-essential. Perhaps it would have been better to go for the term "electives" as used in Ron Harden's SPICES model.

Whatever term is used, the purpose of an elective period of study is to give students an opportunity to pursue personal interests outside the confines of the core course. This may be an opportunity to study in depth some aspect of the core that particularly interests a student, or it may be a chance to tackle a topic that would not otherwise feature at all in the undergraduate course. Not only does the use of elective study allow the course to be broadened to suit individual interests; it also encourages students to take on responsibility for designing their own learning agenda, pursuing new sources of information, and deciding how much they want to learn about a topic.

Like most other strategies, however, electives have their disadvantages. Among other things Ron Harden's group identifies the pressures that staff can experience in trying to coordinate extensive elective programmes for large numbers of students; the difficulties of ensuring adequate supervision for a huge range of topics; problems in motivating staff to get involved in what can be seen as "the students' project"; the danger that, unless timetabling is carefully controlled, electives can interfere with students' attention to the core subjects; and the difficulties in assessing students' performance on electives, given the vast range of agendas set and topics covered.

Systematic curriculum design

The traditional approach to medical education, especially on the clinical course, has been along the lines of an apprenticeship. Students were allocated to a clinical firm and saw patients as they were admitted to the ward. Little overall planning could be done because it was impossible to predict which patients would be available at any given time. The assumption was that students would eventually be exposed to an acceptable range of conditions. Increasingly the acceptability of this approach is being questioned, and in summarising the problems with opportunistic curricula Harden *et al* emphasised the growing feeling that medical schools should be accountable to the public for the quality of the graduates from medical courses.[3] This means that the content of the course cannot be left so much to chance.

The situation is further compounded by increasing specialisation in hospitals. The traditional "general" medical and surgical firms are now few and far between, and the chances that students will see an acceptable range of common conditions during a six month attachment to a hospital firm is much less than previously.

However desirable it may be to introduce some formal planning into the undergraduate experience, it is actually hard to implement a fully systematic approach to medical education. For one thing it is administratively easier to allow teaching to fit in with the way we provide services in our hospitals. While service provision remains essentially firm and specialty based it is hard to provide clinical teaching based on a different structure. (This may, of course, be another reason to look carefully at placing more emphasis on community based teaching, with students attending hospitals only when their own patients do so.)

Another problem about introducing a completely systematic approach is the need to have clinical cases available to illustrate relevant aspects at specific points in the course. Timetabling a section on thyroid disease for a given week is pointless unless suitable patients are available at that time. Two possible solutions are to introduce more cooperation between firms, so that students have access to a wider pool of patients at any given time, and to make more use of simulated patients. These are healthy people who have been trained to mimic the presentation (including physical signs on examination) of specific medical conditions.[16] They are used extensively in North America for undergraduate teaching, but in Britain they are less common.

Implementing curriculum change

The SPICES model illustrates how many factors can be taken into consideration when designing or changing a curriculum. Contrary to popular belief, changing medical curricula is not an "all or nothing" process, and planners should select those approaches that work best in their specific setting. In fact, Ron Harden thinks that "it is inherently unlikely that a position at either extreme end of the [SPICES] spectrum is appropriate." Many innovative schemes in medical education are described in jargon terms that make them sound quite out of the ordinary. But most medical teachers are already using problem based, self directed, small group, and integrated approaches as part of their teaching and doubtless have useful comments to make about when such approaches are helpful. We should ensure that people are not excluded from the current debates because they do not recognise the simple concepts behind the jargon phrases.

1 General Medical Council. *Undergraduate medical education. The need for change.* London: GMC, 1991.
2 Council for National Academic Awards. *Improving student learning.* Oxford: Oxford Polytechnic, 1992.
3 Harden RM, Sowden S, Dunn WR. Educational strategies in curriculum development: the SPICES model. *Med Educ* 1984;18:284-97.
4 Standing Committee on Postgraduate Medical Education. *Teaching hospital doctors and dentists to teach: its role in creating a better learning environment.* London: SCOPME, 1992.
5 Walton HJ, Matthews MB. Essentials of problem-based learning. *Med Educ* 1989;23:542-58.
6 Branda L. Implementing problem based learning. *J Dent Educ* 1990;54:548-9.
7 Neufeld VR, Norman G, Feightner JW, Barrows HS. Clinical problem solving by medical students: a cross-sectional and longitudinal analysis. *Med Educ* 1981;15:315-22.
8 Mitchell DLM, Pallie W, McAuley RG. The simulated tutorial. *British Journal of Medical Education* 1975;9:133-9.
9 Coles CR. Differences between conventional and problem based curricula in their students' approaches to studying. *Med Educ* 1985;19:308-9.
10 Lowry S. Medical education. What's wrong with medical education in Britain? *BMJ* 1992;305:1277-80.
11 Towle A. *Critical thinking: the future of undergraduate medical education.* London: King's Fund Centre, 1991.
12 Lowry S. Medical education. Curriculum design. *BMJ* 1992;305:1409-11.

13 Walton JN. On training tomorrow's doctors: the Newcastle curriculum revised and reconstructed. *BMJ* 1977;i:1262-5.
14 Oswald N. Why not base clinical education in general practice? *Lancet* 1989;ii:148-9.
15 Oswald N. Where should we train doctors in the future? *BMJ* 1991;**303**:71.
16 Stillman P, Swanson DB, Smee S, Stillman AE, Ebert TH, Emmel V, *et al*. Assessing clinical skills of residents with standardised patients. *Ann Intern Med* 1986;**105**:762-71.

Assessing students

Student assessment is often described as "the tail that wags the dog" of medical education. It is seen as the single strongest determinant of what students actually learn (as opposed to what they are taught) and is considered to be uniquely powerful as a tool for manipulating the whole education process. Sir William Osler summed up the power of examinations in 1913: "At the best means to an end, at the worst the end itself, they may be the best part of an education or the worst—they may be its very essence or its ruin."[1] But is assessment as powerful as we think, and, if it is, are most medical educators using it effectively?

Why assess?

Few people formally question why we assess medical students, and many who do think no further than using assessment as a means of checking that required information has been learnt. Certainly in an overloaded curriculum students will pay attention to topics that they know will feature in examinations.[2] A recent study of surgical students at the Flinders University of South Australia (reported by D J Prideaux at the fifth Ottawa international conference on assessment of clinical competence, Dundee, September 1992) found that when no clear guidelines and course objectives were given in a self directed learning programme the students—far from exploring the topic widely and pursuing personal interests—tried to "guess" what would feature in the final examination and concentrated on that. This tendency allows staff to direct students' attention to important topics but also increases the risk that unexamined areas will be ignored.

Unfortunately, the fact that students can successfully answer examination questions on a topic is no guarantee that they will retain their knowledge of the subject. Assessments that are based on a one off, factual recall are notoriously unreliable as indicators of real learning,[3] and if assessment is to be used to ensure learning more complex approaches are needed. One method is to retest the same information at regular intervals. At the University of Maastricht, for example, the entire medical school sits an identical multiple choice "progress test" at various points during the course.[4] This allows students to document their increasing knowledge as they progress through the course and ensures that essential information is not conveniently forgotten once the exam is out of the way.

McMaster University, which has never had formal examinations during the medical course, is now planning to introduce a Maastricht-style progress test. This is largely in response to frequent complaints from students that the complete lack of formal assessment actually adds to their stresses rather than reduces them. Students never quite know whether they have learnt enough about a subject, and it is hoped that a progress test will give them some idea of when it is safe to stop.

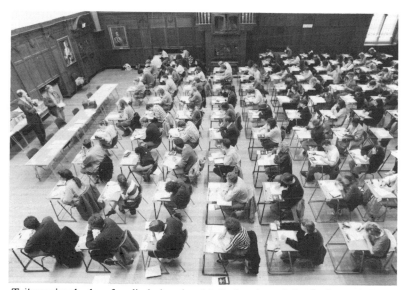

Tail wagging the dog of medical education. Medical students sitting finals at end of their course

Assessment as an aid to learning

An important function of assessment is to aid learning by providing students with a check on their progress and an opportunity to improve. If students are given an opportunity to give feedback to their tutors then assessment can also be useful in refining the way a curriculum is taught and ensuring that course objectives are met. Too often assessment is used purely as a tool for staff to regulate progression of students through the system and rank them in order of achievement.

We tend to rely heavily on summative assessment — testing acquired knowledge at the end of a course (when it is too late to correct deficiencies). Students need formative assessment — regular checks on how they are doing, with detailed feedback on the results and an opportunity to try again after remedial learning. This is a powerful tool in focusing students' learning[5] and can be tailored to individual needs and wants. The Centre for Medical Education, University of Dundee, for example, has devised computer banks of multiple choice questions that students can use as and when they wish to monitor their own progress. Simple feedback can be incorporated into such programmes. More complex feedback may have implications for staff time, but if our aim is to teach rather than to test that must be accepted.

Some medical schools still refuse to provide any feedback on their examinations on the grounds that they need to use the test again the next year and mustn't allow the answers to leak out. A bank of three papers used in rotation should get round this problem, and if that is impossible then by all means hold a summative test without feedback but ensure that separate formative tests are also available. It is inexcusable that many students who have failed an examination are still expected to retake the whole topic with no idea of where they went wrong last time and no guidance on where to focus their attention. That is a waste of their time and is not educational.

Ensuring minimum standards

Because undergraduate medical education is a professional training the minimum standards of professional practice must be acquired during the course. The protection of the public demands this gatekeeping function of assessment, even if it places constraints on the educational experience.

This requirement is universal. McMaster has no summative assessment during the course,[6] but any graduate who wishes to practise medicine must still pass the national licensing exams. Indeed, one criticism often made of the McMaster course is that its students do not do as well as those from other schools in the licensing exams. Dr Barbara Ferrier, a founder member of the medical faculty at McMaster, thinks that this is an oversimplification. For one thing the relative ranking of McMaster students varies from year to year, and over several years no consistent pattern emerges. McMaster students tend to do a bit worse than average on the multiple choice question paper and rather better than average in the patient management section. Secondly, McMaster allows all of its students to enter the licensing exams as soon as they complete the course, whereas many other schools screen out those they think might fail and allow them to enter only after further tuition.

The only sensible way to ensure that minimum standards are met is to define them and fail any student who does not reach them. Why, then, do so many medical schools persist in marking students against their peers rather than against an externally set standard?[7] Most British medical schools use so called norm referenced assessment, in which the students' scores in an exam are ranked on a normal distribution and the pass mark is adjusted to provide a predetermined percentage failure rate. This means that the absolute standard achieved may vary widely from year to year (figure). Because most medical students manage to learn the absolute essentials of a course these basic points have little discriminatory power in a norm referenced examination and are often omitted. The exams thus concentrate on the rarities that will discriminate between the best and worst students, and the basic principles may never be tested.

Norm referenced assessment also raises the possibility that a particularly poor group of students will "pass" the exam despite falling far short of the desired minimum achievement. Conversely, an excellent adaption in the way a course is taught may have dramatic effects on the amount that students learn about a subject, but this will not be reflected in any improvement in the "pass rate."

In criterion referenced assessment, however, the required minimum attainment is determined in advance and students who score less than this standard fail. Norm referenced marking cannot ensure that minimum standards are attained; criterion referenced assessment can. Norm referenced assessment is useful when scores are being ranked before allocation of a limited commodity, such as house jobs,

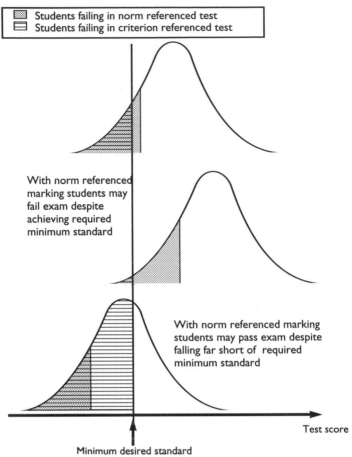

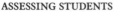 Students failing in norm referenced test
Students failing in criterion referenced test

With norm referenced marking students may fail exam despite achieving required minimum standard

With norm referenced marking students may pass exam despite falling far short of required minimum standard

Test score

Minimum desired standard

Norm referenced marking cannot ensure minimum standards are attained; criterion referenced marking can. Proportions of students failing in the two types of test

but it should not be the main system for assessing medical students' achievements.

What should we assess?

If assessment is so important what should be assessed? Traditionally the emphasis in medical education has been on acquiring a body of essential facts on each topic, but now more attention is given to the skills and attitudes thought to be important in a "good doctor."[8][9] No single examination can be expected to assess such a wide range of features. Medical examiners should identify those aspects that they wish to test and then provide a range of appropriate formats.

There is often a high correlation between students' performance in different types of examination, which has led some people to conclude that they can rely on whatever system is cheap and administratively simple. Professor David Newble of the University of Adelaide, however, emphasises that this correlation may simply be reflecting the relative ability of students to study for exams rather than saying much about their actual knowledge. Most experts now agree that a range of methods is needed to assess a range of clinical skills.[10] The multiple choice question paper, for example, is an excellent, cheap, reliable, and reproducible way of testing factual knowledge but tells us almost nothing about clinical skills. The objective structured clinical examination (box) is expensive, administratively cumbersome, and lacks

---

The objective structured clinical examination

Written papers may be useful tests of factual knowledge but are poor at assessing clinical skills. Traditional clinical examinations are difficult to standardise, and how well students perform may depend largely on the "luck of the draw" in determining who examines them, on which patients, and using what questions. The objective structured clinical examination was devised to provide a more standardised way of assessing clinical competence.[15 16]

- Objectives of the test are identified and recorded. Objective structured clinical examination is then designed to cover all of the required aspects
- Candidates rotate around a series of "stations," at each of which they are asked to perform a clinical task or answer questions on the material provided
- Assessors are present at relevant stations to assess the candidate's performance using a standardised checklist
- Clinical models and simulated patients can be used during objective structured clinical examinations to allow large numbers of students to be tested on the same clinical problem without causing fatigue or distress to real patients
- Marking can be completed as the objective structured clinical examination proceeds and prompt feedback is possible (some centres provide immediate feedback between stations)
- Objective structured clinical examinations can be expensive and administratively cumbersome to set up but are easy to mark and allow testing of skills that more traditional methods ignore

---

McMaster's "triple jump" test

An important aspect of education is learning how to learn. Many medical courses now use large elements of "self directed learning" so that students become familiar with the skills and resources needed to keep up to date with the rapid changes in medical knowledge. The "triple jump" test was devised as a means of assessing students' competence at self directed learning.

- *Step 1:* Student reads the written "problem" and discusses first impressions with tutor. The student then selects some tasks for further learning and decides what additional information is needed
- *Step 2:* During the period of private study the student uses any relevant sources of information to tackle these self selected tasks
- *Step 3:* Student reports back to tutor and presents a revised summary of the problem based on his or her recent researches. The tutor provides feedback on the way in which the student has tackled the problem

---

high reliability but is an excellent way of assessing practical skills.[11-14] Even complex processes like skill at self directed learning can be tested; McMaster has devised the "triple jump" test to do just that (box).[17]

Features of a good test

Given the plethora of techniques for assessing students, there is a real danger of becoming obsessed with the methods and neglecting the content. Professor Cees van der Vleuten, from Maastricht, reminded delegates at the conference in Dundee in 1992 on the assessment of clinical competence that ultimately the care with which any examination is devised is more important than the form that is chosen. What, then, are the cardinal features of a good test?

A good test must be acceptable to those using it, feasible, valid, and reliable. A test may be acceptable to some of those dealing with it and not to others. Multiple choice tests, for example, may be acceptable to those administering them because they are simple to use, cheap to run, and quick and easy to mark. They may be wholly unacceptable to those sitting them if the questions do not seem to be a fair test of the important aspects of a course. A carefully thought out objective structured clinical examination may be a good way to assess essential clinical skills, but the logistic problems of running it may make it unfeasible for the simultaneous assessment of an entire year of students.

A valid test measures what we want it to measure and nothing else. The validity of a test can be assessed under various headings (see box).[18]

Reliability is a measure of the consistency and accuracy with which a test measures what it is supposed to. In a good assessment system not only should the test be reliable but so also should the system for marking it. A multiple choice question paper is usually very reliable and feasible, but because it essentially tests factual recall it may not be very acceptable to candidates and would be unlikely to have high validity as a measure of clinical skills.[19] Essay questions tend to have low reliability (particularly because of difficulties in standardising the marking) and surprisingly low validity. Structured short answer papers have higher validity because more precise instructions can be given to the candidate.[20]

No single examination format will guarantee acceptability, feasibility, validity, and reliability, but care in identifying the strengths

---

Testing terms

Summative assessment: Testing acquired knowledge at the end of a course.

Formative assessment: Regular testing of progress throughout a course.

Norm referenced tests: Scores are ranked on a normal distribution and the pass mark adjusted to achieve a predetermined percentage failure rate.

Criterion referenced tests: Pass mark is predetermined, and the pass rate is allowed to vary with absolute achievement.

Validity: Extent to which a test measures what we want it to measure and nothing else.

Content validity: Measure of whether the test contains a representative sample of the items that we wish to assess.

Construct validity: How well a test measures the feature of interest. (If students do better on a test after studying a course aimed at teaching a particular skill we have some evidence of the construct validity of that test for assessing that skill.)

Criterion referenced validity of a test is judged by assessing how well the test results correlate with another accepted assessment method.

Reliability: Measure of the consistency and accuracy with which a test measures what it is supposed to.

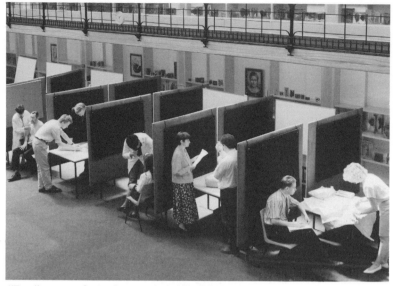

"Excellent way of assessing practical skills." Objective structured clinical examination in progress at St Bartholomew's Hospital, London

and weaknesses of each approach and clear objectives for the assessment should help staff select a useful range of tests.

Criteria for assessment

Assessing medical students should help them focus their learning during the course, identify individual strengths and weaknesses, provide an opportunity for improvement, highlight deficiencies in the content or delivery of the medical course, and, ultimately, protect the public against incompetent graduates. To do all this the assessment system must contain a large and properly managed formative element. The summative assessment must be criterion referenced. There must be adequate feedback between staff and students to ensure that all potential gains are obtained from the assessment system.

1 Osler W. Examinations, examiners, and examinees. *Lancet* 1913;ii:1047-59.
2 Newble DI, Jaeger K. The effect of assessments and examinations on the learning of medical students. *Med Educ* 1983;17:165-71.
3 Tooth D, Tonge K, McManus IC. Anxiety and study methods in preclinical students: causal relation to examination performance. *Med Educ* 1989;23: 416-21.

4 Verwijnen GM, Imbos T, Snellen H, Stalenhoef B, Pollenmans M, Luyk S, *et al*. The evaluation system of the medical school of Maastricht. *Assessment and Evaluation in Higher Education* 1982;3:225-44.

5 Ende J. Feedback in clinical medical education. *JAMA* 1983;250:777-81.

6 Pallie W, Carr DH. The McMaster medical education philosophy in theory, practice and historical perspective. *Med Teach* 1987;9:59-71.

7 Turnbull JM. What is . . . Normative versus criterion-referenced assessment? *Med Teach* 1989;11:145-50.

8 General Medical Council Education Committee. *Recommendations on basic medical education.* London: GMC, 1980.

9 Towle A. *Critical thinking: the future of undergraduate medical education.* London: King's Fund Centre, 1991.

10 Jolly B, Wakeford R, Newble D. Implications for action and research. In: Newble D, Jolly B, Wakeford R, eds. *Certification and recertification in medicine.* Cambridge: Cambridge University Press (in press).

11 Petrusa ER, Blackwell TA, Rogers LP, Saydjari C, Parcel S, Guckian JC. An objective measure of clinical performance. *Am J Med* 1987;83:34-42.

12 Newble DI. Eight years' experience with a structured clinical examination. *Med Educ* 1988;22:200-4.

13 Malik SL, Manchanda SK, Deepak KK, Sunderam KR. The attitudes of medical students to the objective structured practical examination. *Med Educ* 1988;22:40-6.

14 Roberts J, Norman G. Reliability and learning from the objective structured clinical examination. *Med Educ* 1990;24:219-23.

15 Harden RMcG, Stevenson M, Downie WW, Wilson GM. Assessment of clinical competence using objective structured examination. *BMJ* 1975;i: 447-51.

16 Harden RM, Gleeson FA. Assessment of clinical competence using an objective structured clinical examination. *Med Educ* 1979;13.41-54.

17 Painvin C, Neufeld V, Norman G, Walker I, Whelan G. The triple jump exercise—a structured measure of problem solving and self-directed learning. *Annual Conference on Research in Medical Education* 1979;18: 73-83.

18 Newble DI, Hoare J, Elmslie RG. The validity and reliability of a new examination of the clinical competence of medical students. *Med Educ* 1981;15:46-52.

19 Levine HG, McGuire CH, Nattress LW. The validity of multiple choice achievement tests as measures of competence in medicine. *American Educational Research Journal* 1970;7:69-82.

20 Feletti GI, Engel CE. The modified essay question for testing problem-solving skills. *Med J Aust* 1980;i:79-80.

Teaching the teachers

No proper review of an education system should ignore the role of the teachers. But in medical education the teachers are not easy to define. Many current debates about the future of medical education are going on among small groups of specialists, with no input from the vast majority of people who do the actual teaching. Many of the discussions are couched in educational jargon that effectively excludes many "jobbing doctors" who do so much of the teaching.

Medical teachers in Britain may be divided into three main groups: a tiny minority who are trained in educational theory and methods (who often are not medically qualified themselves), staff holding official "teaching" appointments but without formal teacher training, and NHS doctors who teach (in effect, most NHS doctors). Very few medical teachers have had any formal training in teaching methods or educational theory, but in this respect medicine is little different from most university courses in Britain. Medicine differs from many other professions, however, in the huge amount of teaching expected from all of its practitioners. This principle is enshrined in the Hippocratic oath and emphasised in the new contracts for NHS consultants, all of which incorporate a teaching commitment.[1]

Can anyone teach?

This tradition that teaching is part of being a doctor rather assumes that everyone can and should teach. It is not an attitude that would carry much weight in other educational circles, but it is easy to see its roots in the traditions of apprenticeship to a trade. The medical adage

"See one, do one, teach one" is perilously close to the mark, but Dr Jolyon Oxley, from the Standing Committee on Postgraduate Medical Education, thinks that such a system has some merits. In medical education there is a potential conflict between the desire to provide a broad educational experience and the need to ensure a technical training in how to be a doctor. Oxley emphasises that the technical aspects are best taught by the people who do the actual job—"learning at the master's knee."

But there is growing consensus that the broader functions of a medical education, which are assuming greater importance in the undergraduate curriculum,[2] are not so easy to learn from someone untrained in educational method. The Committee of Vice Chancellors and Principals of the Universities of the United Kingdom has recently called for more training in educational methods for all university teachers.[3] A national inquiry into the problems in medical education organised by the King's Fund identified the need for "professional expertise in curriculum development, teaching methods, and assessment" and for opportunities to be provided for regular training of academic staff,[4] and Ron Harden and colleagues have identified staff development courses as an essential prerequisite for the successful introduction of major curriculum reforms.[5]

If doctors are to provide broad educational experiences for their students they must be trained to do so. Facilitating adult learning and developing self direction in students are skills in their own right. In a recent survey, 79% of consultant staff supervising preregistration house officers in Yorkshire admitted that they had had no training in educational method, yet three quarters stated that they would like it.[6]

What are the barriers?

Most doctors claim to enjoy teaching and want to do it well, but various obstacles to good teaching exist in our present system.

"I swear by Apollo the physician . . . that by precept, lecture, and every other mode of instruction, I will impart a knowledge of the Art to my own sons, and those of my teachers, and to disciples bound by a stipulation and oath according to the law of medicine. . . ."

—Hippocratic oath

Perhaps the most obvious is pressure of time. Few people are full time medical teachers, and service requirements, management responsibilities, audit, and research all compete with teaching for staff time. One respondent in the Yorkshire survey summed up the difficulties: "One has to recognise that the pressures on consultants are increasing steadily—workload, management, teaching, financial control, reduction of juniors' hours. . . . Consultants are bound to fall down on one of these."

This conflict of interests would not be so bad if teaching was seen to have an equal claim with the others on doctors' time, but too often it is pushed into last position in the list of priorities. This was clearly identified in the consensus statement from the King's Fund: "Until teaching is recognised to be an important professional activity (comparable in status to clinical service, research and management) it is unrealistic to expect those involved to devote the necessary time and effort to planning and implementing any new curriculum."[4]

During my researches for this series I did not meet a single person who thought that teaching excellence receives adequate recognition in the medical world. No doctor could hope to be appointed to a job or advance his or her career, even in a so called teaching hospital, on the basis of teaching skills alone. Teaching experience is often ignored in applications for medical posts.

Assessing teaching quality

The problem of ensuring that teaching receives equal weighting with research and administration is not unique to medicine. The Committee of Vice Chancellors and Principals' report suggested that part of the explanation for paying little attention to teaching skills in appointing university staff is that many people believe that it is hard to measure teaching ability. But the report concluded that undue emphasis is placed on inquiries about research experience in the mistaken belief that it is easier to assess a candidate's research abilities.[3]

The report did, in fact, identify ways in which teaching skills could be assessed. Among other things it suggested that teachers should be assessed on the clarity of their teaching objectives; the quality of their notes, handouts, and visual aids; the quality of their performance in lecturing, fieldwork, etc; the volume and range of teaching they undertake; the range of assessment techniques they use; managerial responsibilities and innovative approaches that they take on; and the number of invitations they receive as guest lecturers and speakers elsewhere.

An interesting experiment was conducted recently at McMaster University to see whether teaching tasks could be quantified sufficiently to form the basis for financial reward.[7] On the assumption that any reward system should be public, consistent, and reflect the values of the faculty, the researchers devised a questionnaire based on paired presentations of 10 common educational tasks. For each pair eight longstanding members of the medical school staff were asked to indicate which task represented the greatest intellectual challenge and which the greatest amount of "hassle." There was remarkable consistency among subjects in the rankings obtained, and also the suggestion that tasks like teaching interviewing skills—which are difficult to recruit staff for—received high hassle scores. The researchers concluded that such an approach might be extended to develop ways of rewarding people fairly for the educational tasks they undertake.

Solving the problem

A pressing need in reforming medical education is to redress the imbalance between teaching, research, and administration. Not everyone can or needs to excel at everything, and unless people are allowed to concentrate on what they are good at we may be wasting valuable resources. The Committee of Vice Chancellors and Principals' report suggests that more flexibility should "allow staff to be used considerably more effectively than under the present system, where research is considered the prime and often only road to reward and promotion and hence staff expect that the balance of their tasks should be broadly the same for all."[3]

At present funds are allocated to universities by the Universities Funding Committee on the basis of the research grants and scientific papers generated by departments. Some attention should also be paid to the amount and quality of teaching that goes on. The inclusion in NHS consultants' contracts of a formal commitment to teaching is a step in the right direction in that it acknowledges that most doctors teach to a greater or lesser extent. Having established that principle, however, we should move on and demand greater flexibility in interpreting that commitment.[8] Within a department it must be possible for people who have particular interests and aptitudes for teaching to take on a greater share of the load. Nor should we expect the very few who do not want to teach to continue to do so when they might be more usefully employed in management, audit, service, or research tasks.

Status for teaching

Allowing doctors to choose whether to spend time in teaching, or research, or management will work only if all of the options are seen to be of equal importance. Colin Coles emphasises the importance of staff development for those who want to pursue teaching interests.[9] He also thinks that we must develop a culture that demands certain standards from all teachers and accords high status to the few who choose to develop their teaching skills further. Reward does not have to be financial—there is already considerable kudos attached to being an examiner for the major postgraduate colleges and faculties, and we should try to find ways of extending such attitudes to other teaching responsibilities. We should develop systems to reward teaching excellence, both on a daily basis and, possibly, through schemes like the merit awards. We must also ensure that teaching is seen to be important, and a simple way to start is to insist that all doctors must document their experience when applying for jobs and that all appointments committees should ask about it.

Jolyon Oxley warns that we must not reach a stage where teaching is done "only by the professional educators." He thinks that it is more important to convince doctors that "teaching" is a broad term and covers much of what they do every day and to ensure that they receive adequate training and support to carry it out well. Even if we encourage some doctors to specialise in medical education, most of the day to day teaching will remain the domain of jobbing doctors. We must ensure that they receive ample opportunities to improve their skills and monitor their progress.

The Standing Committee on Postgraduate Medical Education is due to report soon to the secretary of state for health on how staff in NHS teaching hospitals can be helped to teach better. Among the likely recommendations are the provision of proper staff development courses in teaching techniques; providing protected time and resources for teaching; and better planning, management, and evaluation of teaching methods.[10]

St Bartholomew's Hospital Medical College, London, now insists that all new appointees should attend at least one approved teaching

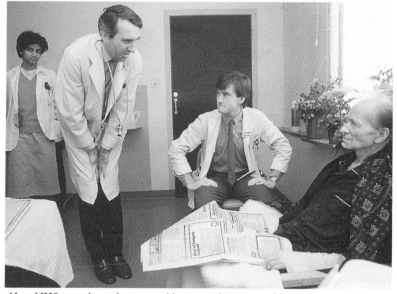

Most NHS consultants have a teaching commitment, yet few receive any training in educational method

course in the year after taking up a post. Although the college makes no further formal demands, staff are encouraged to take part in regular updating courses. Ideally, all doctors should participate in regular ongoing appraisal and training to ensure that they are providing a good service to their undergraduate and postgraduate students.[11 12] The job of training future doctors should be too important to leave to chance.

Sticks and carrots

Colin Coles suggests that the "carrot and stick of reward and reappraisal should be introduced more widely in medical education," with rewards for good teachers and help and, if necessary, penalties for bad ones. Already some medical schools have made progress in implementing such schemes.

In 1978 a committee was established at the University of Washington School of Medicine, Seattle, to develop a programme for evaluating teaching in the school.[13] The committee identified two important functions of such evaluation—to improve teaching and to help to make more informed decisions about staff promotion. The committee's recommendations led to the introduction of formal rating forms on which students graded staff performance in terms of organisation, clarity, and enthusiasm. These assessments were found to have high inter-rater reliability.[14] A system of peer review was also introduced to make qualitative judgments about teaching abilities. Members of staff inform the peer review committee of their teaching responsibilities and of any educational research, staff development courses, or local or national initiatives on teaching that they have attended. A protocol for peer assessment by observing teachers at work was also designed. The scheme, which took three years to devise, is now used in decisions about staff promotion, and since its introduction the average ratings for staff members have improved.

He who pays the piper . . .

Such innovative schemes are not confined to the United States. Dr Helen Pearson, lecturer in medical education at the University of Leicester, has introduced a scheme whereby SIFT money (service increment for teaching; the additional resources provided by the NHS to help offset the extra costs of providing health care in a teaching hospital) is allocated to hospital departments in proportion to the amount of actual teaching that students receive. Students fill in detailed diary records of the teaching each week, recording the setting, time spent in direct teaching, additional time during which students were "learning something" although no formal teaching was going on, grade of the person running the teaching session, etc. Students fill in diaries on a rota basis, with regular cross referencing to check on the accuracy of the entries. In 1991 information was recorded on 3500 student days in the third year alone.

During an introductory lecture the students are reminded that they are entitled to their teaching, and compliance with completing the diaries is high. The data collected allow the medical school to calculate the time actually spent on teaching at each site. SIFT money is then allocated in proportion to the direct costs of teaching in each unit. The scheme was introduced in April 1992 with recommendations to the hospitals about allocation to individual departments. From 1993, however, the departments will receive their money directly, after the fund has been top sliced to pay for the hospitals' infrastructure costs.

The data allow the medical school greater control over the teaching going on in the hospitals. One unit lost over £50 000 when the scheme was introduced, because it was found to be doing much less teaching than had been estimated. Information is also collected about the quality of teaching received, and although this has not yet been formally used in allocating money, one department did have part of its grant withheld for several months until it introduced clear teaching objectives.

Each department takes part in a six monthly review of its teaching quality based on the diary records, and Helen Pearson thinks that eventually the school will be able to move teaching contracts to where the good teaching is. The scheme has made it clear to managers that the teaching contracts represent a substantial part of each hospital's budget, and Helen Pearson says that most managers are now very anxious to work with the medical school to ensure a good service for the students.

Teaching the teachers

Almost all doctors are teachers to some extent—involved in formal or informal training or supervision of students, junior staff, and other professionals. But, perhaps because everyone does it, teaching has a traditionally low status in the medical world. Changes in the sort of education required by students mean that a more professional attitude to teaching must be developed.

We can no longer assume that because someone can do the job they can teach the skill. We must train staff to teach as effectively as possible and should encourage them to see this as an important part of their job. We must also encourage a few enthusiasts to specialise further, taking responsibility for coordinating teaching in their departments. This must be seen as a specialist task, on a par with other administrative duties and research commitments. Proper financial reward should go to those who undertake this important task. Teaching excellence should be rewarded, and there should be real penalties for individuals or units if they fail to fulfil their teaching obligations.

1 Department of Health. *Consultants' contract and job plans.* London: DoH, 1990. (Health circular HC(90)16.)
2 General Medical Council. *Undergraduate medical education.* London: GMC, 1991. (Discussion document by working party of GMC Education Committee.)
3 Elton L, Partington P. *Teaching standards and excellence in higher education: developing a culture for quality.* Sheffield: Committee of Vice Chancellors and Principals of the Universities of the United Kingdom, 1991.

4 Towle A. *Critical thinking. The future of undergraduate medical education.* London: King's Fund Centre, 1991.
5 Harden RM, Sowden S, Dunn WR. Educational strategies in curriculum development: the SPICES model. *Med Educ* 1984;**18**:284-97.
6 Wilson DH. Education and training of preregistration house officers: the consultants' viewpoint. *BMJ* 1993;**306**:194-6.
7 Marrin M. Faculty attitudes toward educational roles in the undergraduate MD program. *Pedagogue* 1991;**3**:1-6.
8 Watson N. Time to revitalise, recognise and reward good teaching—a mid-Atlantic perspective. *Surgery (Abingdon)* 1992;**10**(pt 2):36a-b.
9 Coles C. Education in practice: teaching medical teachers to teach. In: Coles C, Holm HA. *Learning in medicine.* Oxford: Oxford University Press (in press).
10 Standing Committee on Postgraduate Medical Education. *Teaching hospital doctors and dentists to teach: its role in creating a better learning environment.* London: SCOPME, 1992.
11 Irby DM. Clinical teacher effectiveness in medicine. *Journal of Medical Education* 1978;**53**: 808-15.
12 Coles C. Developing medical education. *Postgrad Med J* (in press).
13 Irby DM. Evaluating instruction in medical education. *Journal of Medical Education* 1983;**58**: 844-9.
14 Irby D, Rakestraw P. Evaluating clinical teaching in medicine. *Journal of Medical Education* 1981;**56**:181-6.

The preregistration year

In Britain basic medical education ends with a year as a preregistration house officer in approved hospital posts that provide the general clinical experience required before full registration with the General Medical Council. In theory the preregistration year is an integral part of basic medical education, which is reflected in the fact that the universities have statutory responsibility for this year. But this is also the first time that a young doctor takes on daily clinical responsibility for patients' care, and in reality the service element provided by preregistration house officers underpins the medical care provided in many of our hospitals.

The long hours worked by preregistration house officers, the high service commitment, and the low rating given to the educational aspects of the job have led to numerous criticisms of this part of medical education. Many reports have drawn attention to high levels of dissatisfaction among junior doctors. One survey, conducted in 1986, found that nearly half of the doctors who had graduated in 1981 regretted their choice of career.[1] A recent report by the BMA has confirmed that stress and disillusionment are common among young doctors,[2] and various reports have pinpointed the preregistration year as a time of considerable unhappiness, up to half of preregistration house officers suffering from clinical depression during the year.[3][4]

A common criticism levelled at the preregistration year concerns the long hours of work. Despite recent government initiatives most preregistration house officers still work over 72 hours a week. What causes most distress, however, is not the total number of hours but the inappropriate work expected of junior doctors during this time.[5]

Recent studies have confirmed that large parts of a house officer's week are spent on routine tasks like taking blood, filling in forms, arranging beds for routine and emergency admissions, and filing laboratory reports.[6] The GMC has acknowledged these criticisms in its most recent set of guidelines on what the preregistration year should provide.[7] Universities are supposed to ensure that all posts approved by them for general clinical experience meet the GMC's recommendations. In this chapter I look at what has been proposed by the GMC, whether this can or should be implemented, what the interested parties think about the recommendations, and whether there are any other ways of ensuring that newly qualified doctors are not put off their careers completely before they have properly begun.

What the GMC recommends

In the introduction to its latest guidelines the GMC states that the preregistration year should be "an enjoyable and profitable experience" and calls on the universities to "exercise greater control than hitherto over the duties undertaken . . . the supervision of house officers, the general education provided and the monitoring of house officers' progress." The document sets out various skills that should be mastered during the year and also states that time should be set aside for education, including protected time within the working week for private study. House officers should have named educational supervisors, usually their consultants, who ensure that the educational objectives of the year are met and help with any personal problems that may arise. The educational supervisor is supposed to ensure that the house officer is not "overwhelmed by clinical commitments, overburdened by responsibilities inappropriate to the experience acquired, or undertaking an excessive on-call commitment." The supervisor is meant to undertake, and not delegate, various tutorial functions, including the induction of the new house officer, regular monitoring of progress and assessment of competence, encouraging participation in educational activities, and giving careers advice.

Can it be done?

These may all be worthy aims, but they are so far removed from the reality of most house officers' experiences as to be laughable. How is a consultant physician or surgeon in a busy hospital supposed to find time for the formal educational supervision suggested, much less the pastoral aspects? Who is going to train consultants in the necessary counselling and facilitating skills? Who will provide the cover for house officers attending their education sessions? Is it realistic to expect junior house officers to admit to their consultants that they are overburdened when their career progression depends on getting a good reference? Unless some of these problems can be overcome the GMC's recommendations will be impossible to implement.

A recent survey of 33 consultant staff in Yorkshire found little enthusiasm for the GMC's proposals.[8] Although almost all of them enjoyed supervising house officers, they admitted that there was little formal teaching (as opposed to learning by apprenticeship) and that they had not been trained to provide such teaching. They also thought that pressures from other commitments meant that it would be impossible to provide the sort of supervision recommended or free the house officers to take advantage of the scheme. A typical comment was, "Will somebody tell me who is going to do the work?"

What about a two year preregistration period?

Recently a new proposal for improving the lot of preregistration house officers has been suggested by the Council of Deans of United Kingdom Medical Schools and Faculties.[9] Under this proposal the preregistration period would be extended to two years with first and second year house officers working in pairs, sharing the on call commitment, and providing cover for each other to attend specially structured education programmes. So that the training is not unduly prolonged the deans suggest that the undergraduate course could be shortened to compensate for the extra time spent as a house officer.

Like the GMC's recommendations the deans' suggestion may seem superficially attractive, but it too lacks any semblance of realism about how it might be implemented. No detailed proposals about how the education programmes might be set up are suggested, although the deans concede that they would require "careful thought" and "ingenious timetabling." The additional burden that this would place on other staff is casually dismissed as "to some extent . . . offset by a smaller number of clinical medical students." The NHS is assumed to benefit financially from reduced extra duty payments and reduced medicolegal costs as junior doctors would be "better supervised and less exhausted." This assumption of improved supervision is put forward as a great strength of the proposals, but in fact what is being

61

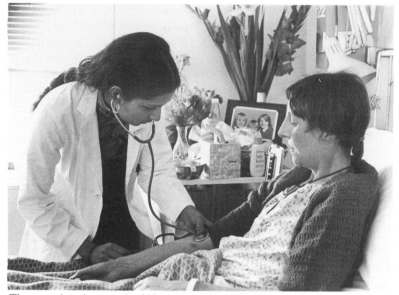

The preregistration year should be an enjoyable and profitable experience. But does it come up to scratch for educational value?

suggested is that the first year house officers would receive supervision from second year staff who are not yet fully registered.[10] There is no discussion about who should provide the improved supervision to the second year staff.

Junior doctor abuse

A recent report from the South Western district based on in depth interviews with 12 preregistration house officers and the staff who had supervised them during their house jobs identified many of the problems with our present system.[11] The report confirmed that house officers spend much of their time on inappropriate tasks—either those that are beyond their competence and for which they cannot hope to provide optimum care (like providing the main source of symptom control to inpatients, the sole medical cover to surgical patients, and explaining complicated procedures to patients and relatives) and others that could be done just as well by non-medical staff (like filing reports, taking routine blood samples, and arranging beds).

There was hardly any educational element of the job, and most of the consultants interviewed admitted that they had not read the GMC's recommendations on this. Those who were familiar with them thought that they were unworkable, given the huge volume of other responsibilities on consultant staff, their lack of training in educational methods, and the absence of support services in most hospitals.

Many of the house officers were working long hours without proper medical supervision. They were very isolated from other members of the team because they were essentially ward based, while the more senior staff spent much of their time in outpatient clinics and operating theatres—often in different hospitals. In fact, much of the day to day supervision and emotional support of house officers was provided by the senior nurses on the wards where they worked, yet this role of the nursing staff receives no official recognition. A combination of long hours, isolation, inappropriate work, and poor working conditions adds up to what Dr Sue Dowling, one of the authors of the report, describes as "a syndrome of junior doctor abuse."

Sue Dowling thinks that it is time that we stopped "tinkering at the edges of the problem" of the preregistration year and totally rethought our responses to it. She suggests that there are two elements of the job—the educational and the service— and that neither has been properly thought out. She suggests that the educational infrastructure does not exist at all in our present system but could be provided. The universities could coordinate distance learning packages for their graduates in various hospitals, although this would have funding and manpower implications.

Total rethink

The service elements of the job fall into two categories—those that are routine and mundane and do not need a doctor to carry them out, and those that are essentially the front line services for health delivery in our hospitals. People who challenge the assumption that much of what a house officer does could be done just as well by someone without a medical qualification may be surprised to learn that in Taunton and Cheltenham nurse practitioners are already working as house officers on two surgical firms (box).

Sue Dowling suggests that front line medical services should not be provided by the most junior member of the team working without adequate supervision. She points out that in specialties where the quality of the front line services is a matter of life and death—such

63

Surgical nurse practitioner

Lou Jacobs has been a nurse for 17 years and has over 12 years' experience in intensive care units. She has been working as a nurse practitioner on a general surgical firm at the Taunton and Somerset NHS Trust since August. In previous years her job has been filled by a preregistration house officer.

Her duties differ from a preregistration house officer's only in line with the legal restrictions on nursing staff. She is not allowed to make diagnoses, initiate drug treatment, or certify death. She clerks patients, organises and attends ward rounds, requests investigations, draws up theatre lists, liaises with anaesthetic and nursing staff and general practitioners, helps in theatre, and does all of the other tasks undertaken by the medical house officers on the other firms at the hospital.

Lou Jacobs finds the job stimulating and admits to being surprised by how hard house officers are expected to work. She suspects that she may get rather more exposure to outpatient clinics and theatre sessions than her medical colleagues because they get bogged down on the wards with tasks that she is not allowed to do. She regards these sessions away from the routine work as some of the most interesting aspects of the job and does not think that the mundane elements of a house officer's post could be "dumped" on another person without some such perks to "relieve the boredom."

as intensive care medicine or accident and emergency work—they are not provided by preregistration staff. But she challenges the assumption that services like postoperative pain control or the provision of medical cover to surgical patients should be seen as less important. She believes that if patients and the purchasers who obtain medical care for them began to demand a better quality of front line service, then hospital managers would very quickly do something to improve the tasks undertaken by and supervision given to preregistration house officers.

Implementing change

One of the great problems in achieving any change in the preregistration experience is that no one seems to have the power and the will to do much about it. Although the GMC issues recommendations about what the year should provide, it does not have any means of enforcing these. The legal responsibility for the house officer year rests with the universities, which have shown few signs of willingness to rock the existing boat. (One notable exception is the University of London, which recently issued guidelines on what was acceptable in a house officer's post and warned that jobs failing to come up to standard would not be recognised.[12])

The people with most interest in changing things are the house officers themselves, but individually they are in a very weak position because they all depend on references from their consultants for registration and career progression. Collectively, however, they have considerable power. Recently the junior staff at Southmead Hospital in Bristol found themselves in bitter dispute with the hospital management over the terms and conditions of their employment.[13] By chance there were several mature graduates at the hospital, including one who was about to emigrate. These doctors, unlike so many preregistration house officers, were not prepared to be walked over, and a campaign of industrial action—including the threat that future students might boycott the jobs at Southmead—led quickly to remedial action.

Sue Dowling believes that part of the reason why house officers are often so impotent in hospital politics is that they are essentially migrant labour—rarely in one place for more than six months. Managers do not really see them as part of the assets of the unit. She believes that junior doctors could be empowered by longer contracts and proposes that house jobs should be arranged in one year (or even 18 month) blocks within single or closely linked units, so that the doctors felt and were recognised as an important part of the service provided. A scheme like this is now planned for Southmead Hospital.

Empowering the house officer

The first step in empowering house officers so that change can happen is to ensure that they know what they are entitled to expect from the job. Few house officers have any idea of the contents of the GMC's recommendations on general clinical experience. The GMC should ensure that all final year medical students understand what they can reasonably expect. Ideally there should be a central record of all approved house jobs, detailing the extent to which they meet the recommendations. Such a "good house jobs guide" is proposed in one recent report[11] and could be produced by the GMC or the BMA. House officers also need to know what to do if their job falls far short of the recommended standards. It is unreasonable to expect them to tackle problems through their consultants, although if they had independent supervisors this might be possible.

A better way might be for house officers to take collective action through their trade union representatives, and the BMA should take the lead in providing this service. Managers need to appreciate that house officers are a vital part of the service they provide and an asset that should be protected. Attaching doctors to single hospitals for both of their house jobs might be one way of making them a more obvious part of the system.

1 Allen I. *Doctors and their careers*. London: Policy Studies Institute, 1988.
2 British Medical Association. *Stress and the medical profession*. London: BMA, 1992.
3 Firth-Cozens J. Emotional distress in junior house officers. *BMJ* 1987;**295**: 533-6.
4 Firth-Cozens J. Stress in medical undergraduates and house officers. *Br J Hosp Med* 1989;**41**:161-4.
5 Rees G. Improving preregistration training. *BMJ* 1992;**304**:981.
6 Leslie PJ, Williams JA, McKenna C, Smith G, Heading RC. Hours, volume, and type of work of preregistration house officers. *BMJ* 1990;**300**:1038-41.
7 General Medical Council. *Recommendations on general clinical training*. London: GMC, 1992.
8 Wilson DH. Education and training of preregistration house officers: the consultants' viewpoint. *BMJ* 1993;**306**:194-6.
9 Richards P. Educational improvement of the preregistration period in general clinical training. *BMJ* 1992;**304**:625-7.
10 Bahrami J. Improving preregistration training. *BMJ* 1992;**304**:981.
11 Dowling S, Barrett S. *Doctors in the making. The experience of the preregistration year*. Bristol: School for Advanced Urban Studies, 1992.
12 Richards P on behalf of Council of Deans of United Kingdom Medical Schools and Faculties. Educational improvement of the preregistration period of general clinical training. *BMJ* 1992;**304**:625-7.
13 Fleming C. Staffing dispute in Bristol trust hospital. *BMJ* 1992;**305**:210.

Trends in health care and their effects on medical education

The General Medical Council has recognised for decades that there are problems in medical education, but little real reform has happened. In recent years, however, there have been dramatic changes in the provision of health care services which are having knock on effects on medical education. Some of these forces could be turned to advantage in shaping medical education.

Specialisation

The GMC believes that increasing specialisation within medicine and the development of postgraduate medical education are among the biggest influences on the way we train doctors.[1] Doctors cannot now make a career in any branch of medicine in Britain without taking part in postgraduate medical education. Each specialty is controlled by a royal college or faculty that dictates the required specialist training programme and sets the necessary standards. As a result the undergraduate medical course no longer needs to provide so much detailed factual knowledge about individual specialties. A newly qualified doctor must be able to function as a preregistration house officer and have the skills to take full advantage of postgraduate education.[2] Realistically, the detailed factual knowledge needed to begin specialist training in most disciplines could probably be learnt by a motivated senior house officer in a matter of a few weeks at the start of specialist training.

By removing much of the factual load from the undergraduate curriculum we can clear space for topics like communication skills, teamwork, audit and management, appreciation of scientific method, ethics, information technology, etc. All of these are relevant to modern medical practice and provide the student with the skills needed to continue learning beyond the sheltered confines of the medical school, and their importance is emphasised in the contents suggested by the GMC for the proposed core medical curriculum (box).[1]

Changing role of hospitals

The huge changes in the politics and philosophy of health care that have occurred in recent years and are having knock on effects in medical education were outlined by N Bosanquet at the conference on developing medical education, University of London, June 1991.[3-5] Much more emphasis is now put on epidemiology, the health of populations, health promotion, and preventive medicine. Maintaining health is as important as treating disease. Demographic changes mean that medicine of old age is becoming increasingly important.

Much of our health care is now provided entirely in the community. General practitioners have a formal postgraduate education system of their own, and the roles of other members of the primary care team have developed to provide a huge range of specialist professional services. These trends have been accompanied by changes in the way our hospitals function. For various reasons, including the opportunities offered by new technology, cost considerations, and consumer demands, inpatient stays are becoming less common and much shorter than ever before. This means that hospitals are increasingly unable to provide the experiences needed by undergraduate medical students. Many conditions are now managed entirely in the com-

---

Contents of core curriculum proposed by GMC

- Clinical method, practical skills, and patient care
- Communication skills
- Normal structure and function: human biology
- Abnormal structure and function: human disease
- People in society
- The public health
- Disability and rehabilitation
- Finding out: research and experiment

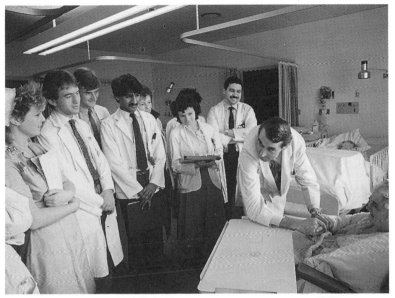

Are teaching hospitals still the best place for undergraduates?

munity or on a day case basis. Fundholding general practitioners are free to negotiate contracts with local hospitals, and many patients with common problems are treated locally and may never reach the teaching wards of distant hospitals. If they do they are often there for only a very short time, during which they may be too acutely ill to cope with the demands of medical students.

The development of minimally invasive investigations and treatments means that much of what goes on in hospitals is inaccessible or irrelevant to students and useful only to postgraduate trainees. If hospitals cannot provide enough suitable patients how can undergraduate students be taught?

Skills laboratories

One obvious response to the shortage of real patients is to develop artificial alternatives. This is not necessarily a second best option. For many professionals—air pilots, for example—simulated situations are an important part of the training programme. The University of Maastricht is famous for its skills laboratory, where students can learn and practise techniques of physical examination, interviewing skills,

69

and invasive procedures without causing undue stress to patients or themselves. A skills laboratory may contain anatomical and clinical models for practising techniques like venepuncture, suturing, and resuscitation; prosected specimens and prepared slides to illustrate anatomy and pathology; computer based, self directed learning packages; and video equipment for practising interviewing techniques. Ideally these facilities are available to all health occupations, so emphasising the team approach to medical care and helping to remove barriers by encouraging students to learn together.

Many British medical schools are developing skills laboratories. Dr Jane Dacre, of St Bartholomew's Hospital Medical School, London, emphasises their value in allowing early practice of difficult, painful, or embarrassing procedures. Access to skills laboratories should ensure, for example, that the first time a doctor passes a urinary catheter is not in the middle of the night, without supervision, and faced with a distressed patient. Jane Dacre does not think, however, that the models available are yet of such a high standard that they can completely replace real patients in undergraduate training. But she believes that, as the demand grows and schools work more closely with the manufacturing companies to ensure authenticity, undergraduates are likely to receive increasing amounts of their practical experience in skills laboratories.

Simulated patients

Another response to the shortage of real patients is to use simulated ones. In the simplest form these are real patients with stable physical signs who are willing to take part in clinical teaching and examinations and who have sometimes undergone simple training in how to present their problems to students. More usually, however, the term is applied to healthy people who have been trained to reproduce features of real patients. Simple briefing can enable a simulated patient to be used for practice of history taking, clinical examination, and skills like getting consent for surgery and breaking bad news. More extensive training can produce a simulated patient who gives a consistent and convincing presentation of a specific medical condition, often to the extent of reproducing findings on examination. Professor Paula Stillman, of Philadelphia, who has pioneered much of the work on simulated patients, estimates that up to 25 hours of specialist training is needed to produce a simulated patient of this type, and extensive retraining is needed to ensure that the performance remains consistent. Simulated patients are paid, but none make it their full time job.

Staff and students who are used to dealing with simulated patients claim that they are so convincing that within minutes the encounter becomes "real." Certainly it is possible to send simulated patients unannounced into general practitioners' surgeries and for them to remain undetected by the doctors dealing with them.[6] In North America simulated patients now form a major element of the teaching programme in many medical schools. In McMaster University they are trained to very high standards and are used to teach and assess students' abilities to take histories and perform physical examinations.

One perceived advantage of simulated patients is that they can be used for student assessment as they can be trained to provide consistent, reliable feedback on performance and can be used many times over without the worries of fatigue or distress that may affect real patients (box).[7] Indeed, in the United States the National Board of Medical Examiners has set up a research project to assess whether using simulated patients might provide a realistic and reproducible means of assessing clinical skills in the national licensing examinations, which currently rely entirely on written assessment.

In Britain simulated patients are used in many schools but in more restricted capacities. Real patients with stable signs are commonly

---

Some advantages of using simulated patients

- They are always available, so teaching can be better structured and less opportunistic
- They are less liable to fatigue than real patients and can be used over and over again
- Staff and students can talk freely in front of them
- Student anxiety is reduced
- Complicating and unrelated problems that might confuse a student do not occur
- Simulated patients can adjust their performance to suit students with different levels of experience
- They can be trained to provide feedback on how the student performs

Some of the "problems" that simulated patients overcome must be coped with in real medical practice, so they cannot wholly replace real patients in medical education.

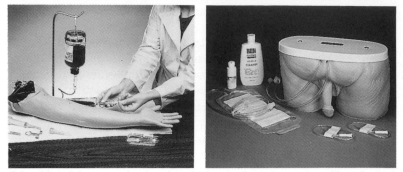

Injectable training arm and male catheterisation simulator. In common with students of other professions, medical undergraduates may gain much experience of procedures by using simulators

used in undergraduate and postgraduate examinations, but usually without any training or modification of their presentation. Inevitably they take no part in marking the students' performances. Several schools use actors to help students learn history taking techniques and explore difficult topics like explaining complicated procedures and breaking bad news. Highly trained simulated patients, used for so much teaching and assessment in America, are essentially unknown in Britain. This is partly because of a reluctance to believe that they can ever replace real situations and partly because of more mundane matters like the expense of training and employing them and the cultural difficulty of persuading healthy British people to volunteer to allow medical students to perform vaginal or rectal examinations on them.

Community based education

Another obvious response to the shortage of suitable patients in our traditional teaching hospitals is to move the students out into the community, where the patients and much of the health care are.[8 9] Several medical schools are developing this approach. Pressure from bed closures led to King's College Hospital, London, transferring one of its general medical firms to the department of general practice for teaching in the community,[10] and Cambridge is to introduce a 15 month community based option for four students as a pilot project in place of their junior medical and surgical attachments and specialty rotations. Although most students in such schemes are attached to general practitioners who act as tutors for the course, community based education is not about studying general practice. It is a way of learning general medical subjects in a new setting. Students study a structured course; they may attend local miniclinics and hospital based outpatient clinics and teaching rounds; patients may be brought up to the surgeries specially for teaching; and self learning packages may be devised for use on the practice computer systems so that students can take full advantage of unstructured time.

Drs Brian Ford and Paul Booton from King's College School of Medicine told a recent conference about the pros and cons of community based education.[10] Among the advantages identified in the experience at King's College and elsewhere are the huge numbers of patients available, the opportunity to see diseases in all stages from initial presentation to recuperation, an understanding of the range of presentations of a condition and the likely differential diagnoses, and the chance to see how illness affects the daily lives of patients and their families (box). Nigel Oswald of Cambridge believes that this gives students a more realistic idea of what medicine is like: "It is more important to see 50 people who might have appendicitis than five who definitely do."

Community based education

Pros
- Provides a realistic response to changes in the provision of medical care
- Overcomes the problem that hospital inpatients present in only one phase of their illness (when they can least help undergraduate students)
- Allows greater availability of patients—most people spend more time at home than in hospital
- Is useful for teaching the core skills outlined by the GMC
- Presents patients in the context of their everyday lives and in proportion to the prevalence of their disease
- Encourages patient centred attitudes
- Encourages self directed learning and self assessment

Cons
- Tutors are fairly isolated and need much training and support
- System is time consuming
- Close relationship between students and tutors may lead to role modelling, which may be good or bad
- May not meet students' expectations of what medicine is all about

---

Among the disadvantages of community based education are the complex planning and administration needed to ensure that all students see an acceptable range of conditions, the fact that rare conditions and extreme complications may not be seen at all, the cost and logistic problems of ensuring that students can follow their patients to clinics and hospital wards as required, and the coordination needed to ensure that standards are maintained when students are taught in small geographically spread groups away from the school base. The practical considerations are numerous. For example, when the Cambridge scheme starts only students who have their own cars will be eligible to take part. Extending such a scheme to an entire school would involve complicated planning of transport, accommodation, and personal safety measures, to say nothing of the academic arrangements. Despite these difficulties Nigel Oswald believes that this approach can and will catch on, and he cites the extensive and highly successful vocational training schemes for general practitioners as evidence of the discipline's willingness and ability to organise large scale, carefully regulated training programmes.

The market economy

Among recent trends that are thought likely to influence medical education is the emergence of a market economy in health care provision. Providers now expect to be paid, and services that are not cost effective may not survive. The introduction of these changes led to fears that teaching would take a back seat in some hospitals as managers emphasised the service elements of doctors' work and tried to balance their books.[3] Teaching medical students has cost implications for hospitals. For example, patients may be admitted earlier than necessary before routine surgery to allow them to be used for teaching while they have physical signs. Extra investigations may be requested or more complicated and experimental procedures used so that students can learn about them. Although the NHS subsidises teaching hospitals through the SIFTR payments for some of the additional costs of providing health care in a teaching setting, there was a worry that market pressures would make teaching hospitals unviable.

In practice, however, things are not as bad as had been feared.[4] Medical schools are slowly recognising that they too are purchasers, controlling substantial sums of money in the form of SIFTR, and that they can negotiate contracts for the type of teaching that they require. A few medical schools, notably Leicester,[11] are already using the placing of their teaching contracts to ensure that hospital managers take education seriously and provide time and resources for it to be done properly.

An opportunity for educators

After years of stagnation medical education in Britain is changing. This is being driven not by educational theory but by the practical implications of technological and political changes. Medical educators must seize this opportunity and take full advantage of these trends. By teaching in a wider range of settings and making more use of simulated situations we can allow students to explore aspects of medicine that are crucially important but difficult to cover in a traditional teaching hospital. We can ensure the best use of all resources by having more to choose from. Students can learn at a more controlled pace and in a more sheltered environment, which may be less stressful to them and to their patients. Changing attitudes to the funding of health care may be the first realistic opportunity that we have had to enforce high standards in medical education.

1 General Medical Council. *Undergraduate medical education.* London: GMC, 1991. (Discussion document by working party of GMC Education Committee.)
2 General Medical Council. *Recommendations on basic medical education.* London: General Medical Council, 1980.
3 Medical Committee of Universities Funding Council. *First report of the effects of the NHS reforms on medical and dental education and research.* London: UFC, 1991.
4 Medical Committee of Universities Funding Council. *Second report of the effects of the NHS reforms on medical and dental education and research.* London: UFC, 1992.
5 Stocking B. *Medical advances: the future shape of acute services.* London: King's Fund, 1992.
6 Rethans JJE, Van Boven CPA. Simulated patients in general practice: a different look at the consultation. *BMJ* 1987;**294**:809-12.
7 Stillman P, Swanson DB, Smee S, Stillman AE, Ebert TH, Emmel V, *et al.* Assessing clinical skills of residents with standardized patients. *Ann Intern Med* 1986;**105**:762-71.
8 Oswald N. Why not base clinical education in general practice? *Lancet* 1989;ii:148-9.
9 Oswald N. Where should we train doctors in the future? *BMJ* 1991;**303**:71.
10 Fine B. Implications of personal tutoring on the community based medical firm. In: Towle A (ed). *Community based teaching.* London: King's Fund, 1992.
11 Lowry S. Medical education. Teaching the teachers. *BMJ* 1993;**306**:127-30.

Making change happen

The problems identified in British medical education are not unique, and many of the proposed solutions have already been implemented elsewhere. Although new medical schools like McMaster in Canada and Maastricht in the Netherlands have had considerable success (in terms of staff and student satisfaction) with courses based on self directed, problem based learning, these models may be dismissed as difficult to implement in an existing course. One example of how major curriculum reform can be introduced into an established and traditional medical course is the recent experience at Harvard.

Harvard's new pathway

Harvard has a reputation as the premier medical school in North America, and the fact that it has chosen to introduce sweeping changes in its course is likely to make other schools take stock of what it is doing. I asked the dean, Professor Daniel Tosteson, why such a successful school had decided to revolutionise its course. Like many recent reforms in medical education the changes had started with the dean's concern at the effects of the traditional course on the students in his faculty. He knew from interviews with students at entry and graduation that many were demoralised by the course. He thought that they were not adequately prepared for their roles as modern doctors.[1] In particular he thought that competence in computer literacy and manipulating information technology, which would help them to be "lifelong learners," were neglected. He was also concerned that the traditional course overemphasised factual knowledge and paid too little attention to the attitudes that modern doctors need to develop towards their patients, their colleagues, and their work.

Seeds of curriculum reform

The traditional medical course at Harvard was a postgraduate entry, four year one with the first two years spent studying the basic sciences and the second two devoted to clinical subjects. The main teaching method was the traditional large lecture. In 1979 the school hosted a "symposium on medical education," which sowed the seeds of curriculum reform in the minds of many of the staff. By 1982 the dean was proposing introducing a "demonstration project" which motivated students could enter (with no specific academic prerequisites) at the end of their second college year. The course would run for seven years, at the end of which graduates would enter the second year of residency programmes. Within the course half the time would be allocated to a compulsory core curriculum and half to self directed learning. Basic and clinical sciences would be interwoven during the course, but with the clinical sciences predominating in the final three years.

A report on these ideas appeared in the medical school newsletter and was picked up by the *Boston Globe* and the *New York Times*. The school soon found itself inundated with applications from college students around the country wanting to enrol on this innovative course.[2] In response to this enthusiasm Tosteson set up a planning group to design an acceptable curriculum for an experimental track within the school.

A major departure from his original vision was the rejection of a seven year course—but other concepts were accepted. The "new pathway" was to emphasise basic concepts rather than facts, topics were to be integrated, and clinical contact was to be introduced early. Initially there was considerable opposition from members of the faculty who feared that the proposals would undermine their own positions. Hence it was decided that the pathway should be set up as a small demonstration project only and be fully evaluated before its concepts were more widely introduced into the school. Guarantees of outside funding from sources including the Josiah Macy Jr Foundation, American Medical International, and Hewlett-Packard also smoothed the introduction of the scheme, which was not seen to present any financial threat to the traditional course.

In the new pathway the formal lecture time was reduced to 60% of

77

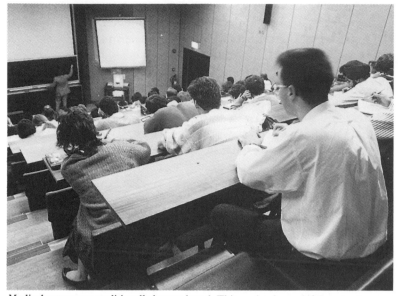

Medical courses are traditionally lecture based. This can be changed if there is adequate funding and an enthusiastic dean

the total available, the remaining time to be used by students to pursue topics that interested them. Most of the teaching was offered in small tutorial groups with close association between staff and students. Formal departmental boundaries were lost, and clinical teachers were involved from the beginning of the course. Each student on the parallel track was given a personal computer to use for electronic mail communication with tutors and other students and for access to bibliographic information. All students were also allocated to a librarian at the library of medicine who would help with the self directed parts of the course.

Evolution of a new system

In 1985 all new students were invited to volunteer to study on the parallel track. Twenty four were randomly selected from the 70 who volunteered. These students were allocated to the "Oliver Wendell Holmes Society" and formed the first group of Harvard students to study under the new system. In 1986, 38 students were enrolled on to the parallel track, but during the next academic year something unexpected happened. Although the original intention had been to formally assess the new curriculum before deciding to extend it to the rest of the school, various forces came into play to ensure that by 1987 the entire 160 strong intake was studying the new pathway course. A major influence was undoubtedly the personality of the dean himself, but the essential catalysts were the decision by the department of anatomy that it could no longer continue to operate two separate curricula—one for the traditional course and one for the parallel track—and the decision by several of the charitable funders of the new pathway that future grants would be available only if the scheme was adopted throughout the school.

The atmosphere within the school was by then receptive to change. The special arrangements that had been made for the new pathway students had caused resentment among other students, who felt that they were being treated like second class citizens, and enthusiasm from staff members who had been involved in the parallel track had reassured other faculty members. Dr Myra Ramos, the associate dean of educational services, thinks that the sudden explosion of the new pathway would have been impossible if Tosteson had been too cautious in his original plans. She believes that any attempt to negotiate an acceptable package for the whole school from the start would have resulted in "minimal change at the margins only." The apparent safeguards inherent in a small pilot project enabled very ambitious changes to be accepted and meant that when the whole school converted to the new programme the change was indeed radical.

One disadvantage of the departure from the planned scheme was, of course, the loss of the opportunity to compare the new pathway students with their colleagues continuing on a traditional course. The new system ran as a parallel track for only two years, and all of the students were volunteers. What evaluation was possible suggests that the new scheme works well. The new pathway students were not identified by tutors in the clinical clerkships, and unreported data collected by Dr Gordon Moore, who coordinated the introduction of the scheme, suggest that new pathway students tended to be assessed as rather better than those who had come through the traditional route. Certainly the first cohort of new pathway students did well in the national board examinations after graduation—but this was a self selected group, who might have done well anyway.

An interesting natural experiment arose when the entire school moved over to the new pathway course in 1987. Students due to enter the school that year had already been asked to volunteer for the parallel track, so two cohorts existed—those who had expressed a preference for the new approach and those who had not. The design of the first year curriculum included mainly a problem based approach, but one course retained a traditional lecture based format. The students' performance on the problem based and lecture courses were not found to correlate with their preference for type of course, and those who had not volunteered for the new pathway did as well as those who had, even on the problem based sections of the new curriculum.[3] Although harder data on the effectiveness of the new approach are not available, there is a feeling at Harvard that staff and students are happier in the new atmosphere. As Myra Ramos told me, "There comes a point where faith and conviction are more important than hard data."

Must change be all or nothing?

Harvard could implement sweeping changes in its medical curriculum because it had a forceful dean and access to large grants to fund a very ambitious project. During my researches for this book I met many people who, though agreeing with the theory behind the reforms of British medical education proposed by the General Medical Council and other bodies,[4 5] do not think that reforms can be implemented on a wide scale. Although schools like St Bartholomew's in London have succeeded in introducing innovative curricula, this is often attributed to the personal skills of the dean and local enthusiasm rather than to anything more generalisable. Can change be introduced in ways that most medical schools would find acceptable?

Colin Coles is a firm believer in change through evolution rather than revolution. He cautions against assuming that the only ways to implement effective reform are to start from scratch (as with McMaster's course, utilising problem based learning in small groups)[6] or to adopt wholesale change as at Harvard. He suggests that the end product of medical education should resemble "a well stocked library capable of updating and cross referencing" and emphasises the importance of "elaborated learning," in which students find that what they learn in various parts of the course "fit together" into a useful, coordinated whole that they can continue to use long after the relevant examination is over.[7]

Although adopting an integrated, problem based course may be one way of achieving elaboration,[8] Colin Coles believes that such radical approaches are not essential. At Southampton, dramatic effects on

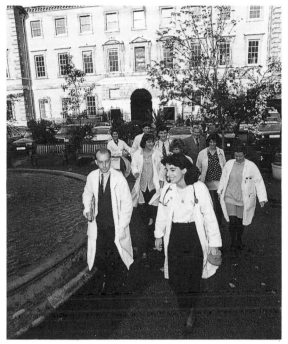

Ultimately the strongest driving force for change in medical education in Britain must be the students and young doctors themselves

students' ability to elaborate have been achieved by changing the timing of their examinations.[9][10] The students sit a traditional 2nd MB examination, which tests their knowledge of basic sciences. But unlike most schools, which set the 2nd MB at the end of the second year of the course, before the students start their clinical studies, Southampton has moved the exam to the end of the third (first clinical) year. The students find that the basic sciences "make sense" when they come to revise them in the light of some clinical experience—as one student said, "It's not so much revision as vision."

Making change happen

The GMC has announced that our system of medical education must change.[4] There is a wide consensus among medical educators and students about the need for change and the direction it should take,[5] and there are plenty of examples from Britain and elsewhere that change is possible and can be effective. But how can we ensure that action results from all of the recent rhetoric? The enthusiasm of

81

staff and students in places like McMaster confirms that techniques like problem based and self directed learning can make medical education an enjoyable experience without loss of quality in the end product. The sweeping changes that have occurred recently at Harvard and the new basic sciences curriculum at St Bartholomew's Hospital, London, prove that change can be implemented in long established, traditional medical schools if there is adequate funding and an enthusiastic dean. The researches into medical education going on at places like Southampton and Dundee confirm that smaller adjustments to medical courses can have useful effects on how students learn. Changes in the provision of health care and increasing awareness of the demoralising effects of our traditional system on the students going through it are driving changes, and we may be poised on the brink of a steep acceleration in the number of schools willing to make radical changes in their courses. But we must ensure that changes are implemented quickly and on the scale needed to address the current problems.

The ultimate responsibility for reforms in medical education rests with the education committee of the GMC. Although the committee is to be congratulated for its lead on the need for change, this will be worthless unless it is willing to ensure implementation of those changes. The GMC does not have a good track record in ensuring that change happens. This is partly because the council has limited means of enforcing its recommendations, short of the draconian removal of recognition from an entire course. If, however, the council is serious about the need for reform it must be willing to find innovative ways of enforcing its recommendations. Although the few schools that have introduced changes seem to be enthusiastic about them, wider implementation will require sticks as well as the nebulous carrots of increased staff and student satisfaction.

Influence of medical students and young doctors

The GMC may have its hands tied in terms of the disciplinary action that it can take, but it is in a position to collect information that could be used by other interested bodies. Mr Richard Wakeford, senior research associate at the University of Cambridge School of Clinical Medicine, has already conducted a series of surveys into educational practices at British medical schools for the council, but the results have not been made public.

Chris McManus suggests that the GMC should routinely collect information from medical students about all aspects of their courses.

This should not be a formal response during the education committee's infrequent assessment visits to a school but should be a regular, in depth assessment of the type of teaching and general experience provided on each course. The GMC is in touch with all final year medical students and house officers when they apply for provisional and full registration, and it would be a simple administrative matter to require applicants for registration to complete an anonymous questionnaire about their educational experiences. This information could be used as the basis of a "good school" or "good house job" guide, allowing students themselves to influence the educational experience by voting with their feet against poor courses.

Ultimately the strongest driving force for change must be the students and young doctors themselves. Individually, medical students and young doctors have little power, but collectively they can be more influential. The falling numbers of applicants to study medicine may force schools to think again about the courses they provide. Recent changes in primary and secondary education in Britain, with increasing emphasis on project work and self direction, may encourage school leavers to seek out courses that continue these approaches. Organisations like the GMC and the BMA should provide students with the information on which to base such choices. Students must be empowered to demand excellence in the courses that they attend and realise that their education is not a favour to them but a means of preparing them to be the sort of doctors that we want in the future.

1 Tosteson DC. New pathways in general medical education. *N Engl J Med* 1990;322:234-8.
2 Ramos M, Moore GT. The new pathway to medical education. In: Kantrowitz M, Kaufman A, Mennin S, Fulop T, Guilbert J, eds. *Innovative tracks at established institutions for the education of health personnel.* Geneva: World Health Organisation, 1987.
3 Moore GT. The effect of compulsory participation of medical students in problem-based learning. *Med Educ* 1991;25:140-3.
4 General Medical Council. *Undergraduate medical education.* London: GMC, 1991. (Discussion document by the education committee of the GMC Education Committee.)
5 Towle A. *Critical thinking. The future of undergraduate medical education.* London: King's Fund Centre, 1991.
6 Neufeld VR, Woodward CA, MacLeod SM. The McMaster MD program: a case study of renewal in medical education. *Acad Med* 1989;64:423-43.
7 Coles CR. Elaborated learning in undergraduate medical education. *Med Educ* 1990;24:14-22.
8 Coles CR. Differences between conventional and problem-based curricula in their students' approches to studying. *Med Educ* 1985;19:308-9.
9 Coles C. The actual effects of examinations on medical student learning. *Assessment and Evaluation in Higher Education* 1987;12:209-19.
10 Coles C. Is problem based learning the only way? In: Boud D, Feletti G, eds. *The challenge of problem based learning.* London: Kogan Page, 1991.

Letters to the Editor, *BMJ*

While the series "Medical Education" was running in the "BMJ" some interesting experiences of those involved in training doctors were published in the correspondence columns of the journal. Some of the letters received up to the time of going to press are published below.

EDITOR,—Having trained in Britain, I am now gaining a Caribbean and American perspective as executive dean of an "offshore" medical school. Stella Lowry asks [pp 1-10] what is wrong with medical education in Britain.[1] The problem seems to be not with medical education, the curriculum, or the teachers but with the structure of the medical schools. In a closed system they have grown used to having many applicants for few places. The future and performance of their graduates are of no concern to them. House jobs and higher posts are all largely in their gift. I think that this has played a large part in the disillusionment of newly qualified doctors and the loss of interest in medicine as a career among school leavers.

The situation at Ross University Medical School, an offshore school for American citizens, is different.

The goal of the basic science campus is to prepare our students for the United States medical licensing examinations—specifically, step 1. If our pass rate is low we will have difficulty attracting students, getting federal loans for them, and finding American hospitals in which they can do their clinical rotations. If our students do poorly in their clinical rotations we will have difficulty placing further students in that hospital. The better their scores in the United States medical licensing examination, the better the residencies they will obtain. The better our graduates do in finding residencies and fellowships, the better students we can attract to the school. The performance of our students is crucial to the school's survival.

Britain does not have a comparable system. There is no national examination. External examiners from another school merely perpetuate the cosy status quo, whereby what happens to graduates and their quality are of little interest to the schools.

If the General Medical Council administered a national licensing examination and the schools' results were published then the schools would be more purposeful and concerned. The council would also have a chance to influence the quality and scope of medical education.

PHILIP COOLES

Ross University Medical School,
PO Box 266,
Roseau,
Commonwealth of Dominica,
West Indies

1 Lowry S. What's wrong with medical education in Britain? *BMJ* 1992;305:1277-80.

EDITOR,—Medical student selection is a difficult area in which to introduce change, but Stella Lowry's article [pp 11-18][1] was too nihilistic.

The argument advanced—that there are so many and varied opportunities after graduation that selectors should not agonise too much about choosing the "right sort" of candidate—is the height of complacency. Companies invest large sums of money in selecting the right people because it makes good business sense.

The author acknowledges that selecting medical students has more lasting implications than for other university courses. The fact that it is difficult does not mean that we should not strive to improve it.

In 1989 Alan Porter and I pointed out that very little of the information on an UCCA form (the only shortlisting information available) has predictive validity for clinical performance.[2] Results at A level are usually only predicted; the head teacher's report is hardly impartial; and the applicant's "interests" are often tailored as a result of coaching by careers teachers. Medical students are often immature and ill prepared for the traumas of medical training, as illustrated recently in the television series *Doctors to Be*.

One immediate partial solution would be to permit application only after completion of A levels. Applicants would be more mature and have an opportunity to show the use to which they had put the available time. The A level results would be real rather than predicted. Motivation towards being a doctor would be tested by the enforced year's delay. It has the added advantage of zero cost. Implementation would clearly have to be phased.

Further research into the predictive validity of a whole range of information would be useful. Biographical details (biodata) have been shown to be useful in some studies in the United States.[3-6] Selection by desired learning styles is of interest, but should wait until we have achieved desired teaching styles.

GEOFF ROBERTS

Camberley,
Surrey GU15 2HJ

1 Lowry S. Student selection. *BMJ* 1992;305:1352-4.
2 Roberts GD, Porter AMW. Medical student selection: time for change. *J R Soc Med* 1989;82.288-91.
3 Ambrosino RJ, Brading PL. An analytical computer-based methodology for screening medical school applicants. *Journal of Medical Education* 1973;48:332-5.
4 Best WR, Diekema AJ, Fisher LA, Smith NE. Multivariate predictors in selecting medical students. *Journal of Medical Education* 1971;46:42-50.

5 Haley HB, Juan IR, Paiva RE. MCAT scores in relation to personality measures and biographical variable. *Journal of Medical Education* 1971;**46**:947-58.
6 Rabinowitz HK. A program to recruit and educate medical students to practice family medicine in underserved areas. *JAMA* 1983;**249**:1038-41.

EDITOR,—Stella Lowry concludes her article on student selection [pp 11-18] by saying that "we must encourage more applicants by reversing recent negative images of medicine as a career."[1] As long as this government is intent on a market led society, fundholding, hospital trusts, and two tiers of medical care is it surprising that candidates who are caring and have the "right" attitudes to enter medicine are now shunning the profession?

I entered medical school in 1961, an idealist and great supporter of the NHS principle that good health care is for all and independent of a patient's means. I still believe that the whole community should be able to have access to the best care. Unfortunately this is not so. I recently found out that a patient of mine could not undergo coronary artery bypass grafting because the health authority had spent its allocation for this operation—a decision made by an administrator who did not take into consideration the patient's clinical needs. Is this progress? Is this the NHS that the country wants? I am sure not, and that is why students are looking elsewhere for job satisfaction.

B OLSBURGH

Health Centre,
Whitley Bay,
Tyne and Wear NE26 2ND

1 Lowry S. Student selection. *BMJ* 1992;**305**:1352-4.

EDITOR,—There is a general perception that change in medical education is starting to occur. It may be difficult for a medical school, itself relatively small, to plan and implement this. The City and East London Confederation for Medicine and Dentistry consists of Queen Mary and Westfield College, the London Hospital Medical College, and St Bartholomew's Hospital Medical College. Cooperation between their staff and students has been extremely effective in providing a critical mass for generating ideas and implementing new teaching methods.

The students of Queen Mary and Westfield College (not of St Bartholomew's as stated in Stella Lowry's article [pp 19-26][1]), which is next to the Royal London Hospital (Mile End), undertake at Queen Mary and Westfield College the innovative phase I of the curriculum which Lowry describes. This is taught by staff of all colleges including basic and behavioural scientists, clinicians, and community staff. The educational content of all phases is supervised by the curriculum management committee of the City and East London Confederation, on which the three colleges are represented, and to which all local implementation groups are responsible. During phase II (in which behavioural sciences, statistics, ethics and the law, and clinical and communication skills are taught, and further project and community experience is gained), the students go to their "parent" medical colleges (the London or St Bartholomew's colleges).

The main clinical modules constitute phase III, and their aims and teaching methods are carefully scrutinised by the phase III committee to ensure suitability and avoidance of factual overload. This committee, again, includes members of all three colleges and incorporates clinicians, basic and behavioural scientists, and students. Such cross college and interdisciplinary pressure has been found invaluable in replacing passivity and resistance to change by enthusiasm and a desire to innovate and improve.

The modules in each medical college are similar but utilise local strengths to best advantage. For students at the London Hospital Medical College the "core" attachments will be supplemented in their final year by two months of electives and three months for the study of more strictly defined "options."

There is a point of particular concern. The cheapest and easiest way of teaching subject matter is by large group lectures. The cheapest and easiest way to teach clinically is by apprenticeship. These are educationally unsatisfactory and unlikely to generate the deep thinking referred to by Lowry or produce caring doctors with a holistic attitude to illness and their patients. Good education is not cheap, as we have already found, and meeting the ideals of the General Medical Council is more costly and time consuming than older methods of medical education.

F P MARSH

The London Hospital Medical College,
University of London,
London E1 2AD

1 Lowry S. Curriculum design. *BMJ* 1992;305:1409-11.

EDITOR,—The logistic problems that Stella Lowry associates with community based teaching [pp 27-39][1] could be resolved by funding in proportion to that supporting teaching hospitals.[2]

Such teaching is certainly feasible. As distinct from the four week experience of general practice which all of our final year students receive (with a final objective structured clinical examination (OSCE) in general practice) this university department of general practice has over many years provided generic clinical teaching for the department of medicine.

In year 1, all 130 students now have four introductory sessions—dealing with people, professional ethics, problem solving, and population based medicine—at local practices. General practitioner tutors are paid at NHS consultant rates for both teaching and training sessions. Patients' expenses are reimbursed and buses are hired for students. The total cost is about £100 per student. This is a realistic estimate of the cost of "casual" systematic teaching. Major resources and imaginative mechanisms[2] are, however, required to enlarge the scale.

The infrastructure of teaching hospitals is largely NHS (rather than university) funded and there has only recently been a welcome extension of this mechanism to general practice. Including this, the combined funds in my region are about £20m a year for hospital as against £0·3m for general practice. Per student per year, general practitioners' funding is about 50% of the hospital rate. These differences merely reflect the current balance of locus of academic activity and the obviously higher unit costs of hospital infrastructure.

General practice based education is still a marginal activity. Even modest expansion will need funds to provide accommodation and resources for good systematic teaching and protected academic time through enhanced staff levels.[2] Our vision should not be clouded by present logistic and structural constraints: the NHS reforms have shown how quickly these can be changed. Although a fivefold increase in funding for academic general practice may seem inconceivable, it is a comparatively modest sum that would drive change in the balance of clinical education and pay handsome dividends for both the patients and the profession as a whole.

ROSS J TAYLOR

Department of General Practice,
University of Aberdeen,
Aberdeen AB9 2AJ

1 Lowry S. Strategies for implementing curriculum change. *BMJ* 1992;**305**:1482-5.
2 Taylor RJ. General practice in the medical school: the way ahead. *Update* 1985;**30**:615-8.

EDITOR,—Stella Lowry offers some profound insights into the problems, current and long standing, in medical education. We are particularly struck by the concern that doctors are now expected to work in multidisciplinary teams, not automatically as their leaders.[1]

To respond to this development in a positive way, in Southampton we have introduced multiprofessional teaching for students from physiotherapy, occupational therapy, nursing, podiatry, and medicine. Problem based learning techniques are used, and students work in teams to define professional roles and develop management plans for patients.

Feedback suggests that students enjoy the experience, acquire knowledge about professional roles and patient management, improve their teamworking skills, and develop positive attitudes towards multidisciplinary teamworking which might serve them well in their later professional practice. As facilitators, we have also learned a great deal about our professional roles.

If medical education is to respond to modern developments in health care, we believe that more of this sort of teaching will be required.

I PHILP	C GALLAGHER
V POMEROY	A ADAMS
	C GRIFFITHS

Faculty of Medicine,
University of Southampton,
Southampton General Hospital,
Southampton SO9 4XY

1 Lowry S. What's wrong with medical education in Britain? *BMJ* 1992;**305**:1277-80.

EDITOR,—The recent articles by Stella Lowry[1][2] have highlighted several important issues in medical education arising from the recommendations of the recent GMC report.[3] At Manchester University, "core plus option" curricular changes have already been implemented. Most traditional style, discipline oriented lectures have been discontinued. We anticipate that our integrated clinical practice course will encourage students to adopt a more holistic approach. The new "option" teaching gives each student the opportunity to study a particular area of interest in depth, and may well influence their final career choice. We hope that the enthusiasm and effort that we are investing in these options will be reflected in the recruitment of graduates into obstetrics and gynaecology.[4]

To complement these curricular changes the nature and timing of the examinations have been changed. Students receive their "core" teaching in the fourth year, with a clinical examination in each core specialty. In obstetrics and gynaecology we have implemented an objective structured clinical examination (OSCE). Lowry highlighted the organisational problems associated with such examinations [pp 40-49].[2] We have overcome these problems and now have what we consider to be a much fairer and more objective examination. The examination (for each group of 90 students) starts at 9 am, and by 6 pm the final results have been confirmed at the examiners' meeting. We have identified the "core" skills which we feel are essential—these include communication skills assessed by history taking, and obstetric and gynaecological examination (the latter using a dummy). We have incorporated written short answer questions and clinically oriented slides.

The marking of the examination is weighted towards the assessment of clinical skills. The final result awarded to each candidate takes into consideration the formative assessment results obtained during their clinical attachment, which incorporates a summative assessment obtained before the examination. A criterion referenced marking schedule is used to assess the students at each clinical station. We use a norm referenced method on the cumulative result to identify those students who require further tuition in our discipline. Any student who fails the examination has a compulsory revision "option" in final year. Students who do not achieve a satisfactory pass in the fourth year have a formal clinical examination and viva during their final MB examination. The final MB now consists of three integrated papers: multiple choice questions, slides with short answers, and a paper consisting of patient management problems encompassing all disciplines.

The new curricular teaching and examinations are very labour intensive and have considerable resource implications. University departments operating within close margins with respect to staffing and clinical resources have to rely on a large measure of good will to achieve continued high standards in teaching and evaluation, which can be difficult to sustain if, for example, reappointments of staff are delayed. Proposals for resource allocation according to quality of teaching as well as research endeavour are undoubtedly overdue.

P J DEWART
MAX ELSTEIN

Department of Obstetrics and Gynaecology,
University Hospital of South Manchester,
Manchester M20 8LR

1 Lowry S. Curriculum design. *BMJ* 1992;305:1409-11.
2 Lowry S. Assessment of students. *BMJ* 1993;306:51-4.
3 General Medical Council. *Undergraduate medical education. The need for change.* London: GMC, 1991.
4 Elstein M. Undergraduate education and recruitment in obstetrics and gynaecology. *Eur J Obstet Gynecol Reprod Biol* 1991;41: 37-42.

EDITOR,—In her article "Teaching the teachers" [pp 50-58] Stella Lowry points out that few medical teachers in Britain have any formal training in educational skills or theory.[1] Since so few doctors possess such skills, perhaps we can learn them from teachers outside the medical profession (at least until there is a sufficiently large body of trained teachers within the profession).

One possibility is the City and Guilds course 730, the further and adult education teacher's certificate. This course is very widely available and it is pitched at the right level for the medical teacher. It is taught in colleges of further education and polytechnics (now universities) throughout the country. (In London, courses are listed in *Floodlight*.[2]) The first term, part 1, covers lesson planning and presentation skills. It would be suitable for any doctor, even if he or she does not specialise in teaching. The remaining two terms cover the basic theory of education and teach how to plan an effective educational programme. This would be ideal for any doctor who wished to be a clinical tutor, or who had a special interest in education.

When I did this course (in 1988 at Lewisham College) I went to tutorials for three hours twice a week, at which theory was taught, and we engaged in teaching exercises assessed by our peers and tutors. There was, in addition, supervised teaching practice in the workplace. We were expected to plan, implement, and evaluate a short teaching programme. There was also a considerable amount of written work, with six written or practical assignments in the first term and a further 16 assignments in the rest of the course. Anyone interested in the content and level of the course may wish to refer to one or more of the texts listed below.[3-5]

I would, however, sound a note of caution. It seems to me that the time, effort, initiative, and determination required to complete this course are equivalent to what is needed to complete a research project. As Lowry points out, teaching does not have the same status as research. The certificate has counted for little in my appointment interviews, and I was repeatedly told after failing the interview that my research record was weak. Until the status of teaching improves in the medical profession it seems unlikely that doctors in training will choose to make the efforts necessary to acquire teaching skills.

BILL PLUMMER

Department of Psychiatry,
United Medical and Dental Schools,
Guy's Hospital, London SE1 1NP

1 Lowry S. Teaching the teachers. *BMJ* 1993;306:127-30.
2 *Floodlight. London's guide to part time day and evening classes.* London: Association of London Authorities, London Boroughs Association, 1992.
3 Curzon LB. *Teaching in further education.* 4th ed. London: Cassell, 1990.
4 Minton D. *Teaching skills in further and adult education.* London: Macmillan, 1991.
5 Newble D, Cannon R. *A handbook for medical teachers.* 2nd ed. Lancaster: MTP Press, 1987.

EDITOR,—Stella Lowry's article describing many ways of improving the preregistration year [pp 59-68] is thought provoking.[1] She mentions that Southmead Hospital is considering changing to a one year block contract as a means of empowering house officers and helping them to be recognised as an important part of the service provided. Some of the stimulus for this came from a survey of senior medical students, yet when 30 current house officers were consulted all but two said that, though they would be happy to have the opportunity to apply for both jobs at one hospital, they would not have applied for a one year block contract that restricted them to one hospital. The ability to gain experience in different hospitals was seen as an important part of the preregistration year, and one year block contracts could limit this.

We should be careful to avoid introducing change for change's sake and should carefully evaluate potential disadvantages as well as advantages. Southmead Hospital has an excellent induction and core curriculum educational programme, which could be coordinated regionally or nationally; it also organises regular trouble shooting meetings between lead consultants, managers, and all levels of junior medical staff. These measures alone may be as effective a means of recognising house officers as an important part of the service provided as restricting them to one hospital site for their preregistration year.

JOHN HARVEY

Southmead Hospital, Bristol BS10 5NB

1 Lowry S. The preregistration year. *BMJ* 1993;306:196-8.

EDITOR,—Stella Lowry[1] underplays a striking finding of David Wilson's survey of 33 consultants in Yorkshire: he found that consultants generally did not see the preregistration year as an educational process.[2] This is remarkable as the universities have a statutory responsibility for this year and it is an integral part of medical education that is required before full registration with the GMC.

I know many consultants who take supervision of preregistration house staff seriously, scheduling regular meetings and teaching sessions and using checklists to ensure that skills and techniques are mastered, but it seems that these consultants are in the minority.

We are now entering the era of strict personal accountability, value for money, and survival of the fittest. In this atmosphere one assumes that consultants who fail to educate preregistration house officers will lose the privilege of having such a colleague.

JAMES D WALKER

Department of Laboratory Medicine and Pathology,
Medical School,
University of Minnesota,
Box 198 UMHC,
Minneapolis, MN 55455-0385,
USA

1 Lowry S. The preregistration year. *BMJ* 1993;306:196-8.
2 Wilson DH. Education and training of preregistration house officers: the consultants' viewpoint. *BMJ* 1993;306:194-6.

EDITOR,—In her series on medical education Stella Lowry has failed to mention one major initiative in community based medical education. The department of primary care at University College London Medical School has been running a community based general medical firm for first year clinical students since September 1991. This six week firm has replaced one of the traditional hospital based medical firms. The model that we have developed is to attach students in pairs to a general practice tutor in a teaching practice. The students spend half the week in the practice, where they see patients at home or in the surgery. They are expected to take a full medical history and perform a physical examination. Once they have finished they are joined by their tutor, who goes through the history and supervises their examination skills.

The programme is structured, and tutors are asked to ensure that students see patients with problems pertaining to the "topic of the week." These topics are chosen to reflect prevalent clinically important medical conditions—for example, ischaemic heart disease, diabetes, asthma and chronic obstructive airways disease, common cancers, and stroke and other common neurological conditions. At the end of each week there is a plenary session on the topic of the week, in which students present patients they have seen and reflect on what they have learnt. The programme is problem oriented and concentrates on teaching the core clinical skills of history taking, physical examination, and communication with patients. The department also runs seminars on developing clinical and communication skills to reinforce the students' experience in the practices.

Students find the firm both educational and enjoyable; in particular they appreciate the one to one teaching from the general practice tutor and the structured nature of the firm. The programme developed from a pilot study with four students per firm. This academic year the number of students per firm has increased to eight and we are collaborating with the department of oncology at the Whittington Hospital, which undertakes a fifth of the teaching. Next year we intend to have two parallel firms of eight students each. This will account for half the 215 students in the year, and we hope to continue expanding until all first year students participate in one community based general medical firm.

ELIZABETH MURRAY   VIVIENNE JINKS
ANDREW HAINES   MICHAEL MODELL

Department of Primary Health Care,
University College and
  Middlesex School of Medicine,
Whittington Hospital,
London N19 5NF

1 Lowry S. Trends in health care and their effects on medical education. *BMJ* 1993;**306**:255-8.

EDITOR,—Dr Nigel Oswald, cited by Stella Lowry,[1] is correct in implying that learning skills in clinical decision making requires seeing large numbers of patients in a short space of time. This, however, is an argument against rather than for community based learning.

This is illustrated by an example from our practice. An average general practice of 10 000 patients refers 34 patients a year for assessment of breast lumps. A student attending a well directed breast clinic may personally see this number of patients in less than a month and be taught to make an accurate clinical assessment. She or he would have to spend a year in general practice to have the opportunity to acquire similar skills. To paraphrase Oswald, "It is more important to see 30 patients who might have breast cancer than five who do (but it is useful and likely that you will see them too)."

DAVID HOCKEN
DAVID GERRARD

Breast Clinic,
Department of Surgery,
St Bartholomew's Hospital,
London EC1A 7BE

1 Lowry S. Trends in health care and their effects on medical education. *BMJ* 1993;306:255-8.

EDITOR,—In her review of methods of assessing students [pp 40-49] Stella Lowry argues the need for methods of assessment that match learning objectives.[1] Considerable advances have been made in the assessment of knowledge and clinical skills—for example, multiple choice questions and objective structured clinical examinations. In addition to providing the knowledge and skills needed for medical practice, the new curriculum at the medical schools of the Royal London Hospital and St Bartholomew's Hospital aims to foster lifelong learning and awareness of strengths, weaknesses, and learning needs. As a part of this the development of skills in self reflection and self critique of performance is important for continuing learning and personal development.

A new formative assessment for third year students has been introduced this year—namely, an integrated workbook assignment. This entails interviewing a patient, tape recording the interview, selecting a section to transcribe, and analysing the communication process involved in taking the history. The student must also write up the medical history and examination findings and discuss the psychosocial, ethical, legal, and nursing considerations of the patient's case. This task, which follows on from a programme covering these subjects, incorporates the strands of communication skills, behavioural sciences, ethics, and law in the assessment. Students must complete a satisfactory workbook assignment before entering parts 5 to 10 of the MB BS examination.

To overcome the problem of case specificity, assessment of the interview section is based not on how well the students did but on their ability to evaluate their communication with the patient. Their critique is verifiable by reference to the tape recording of the interview. Students do not have to search for the "ideal" patient. Even if they were not satisfied with their history taking, their analysis of their performance, the difficulties or constraints perceived, and ideas for improvement are the most important material for assessment in this task.

The first cohort of 240 students has just completed this assignment. The students have reported useful insight from their self assessments and have been able to identify things they did well, problems, and how they could improve.

This method of assessment matches two key aims in our new curriculum. Firstly, in relation to the communication skills part it addresses the development of students' skills in self awareness and reflective learning. Secondly, the workbook encourages the students to understand their patient as a complex person whose health and wellbeing depend on more than biomedical considerations. The depth and extent of this understanding have been shown in some work of exceptional quality and insight.

We believe that the integrated workbook assignment embodies the ideals of our curriculum and, in particular, has considerable potential for continuing the General Medical Council's recommended strands of ethics, law, behavioural science, and communication skills throughout the clinical course.

ANNIE CUSHING
LEN DOYAL
PETER HAJEK
SHEILA HILLIER

Confederation of East London Colleges,
London Hospital Medical College,
London E1 2AD

1 Lowry S. Assessment of students. *BMJ* 1993;306:51-4.

EDITOR,—As one who taught on Harvard's "new pathway" during the two pilot years,[1] as well as on its traditional courses, I would like to make some comments.

The success of any programme rests on the faculty's enthusiasm and support. Teaching well takes time and often yields little tangible reward. Harvard's new pathway got through its pilot years relying on the motivated staff and fellows. This staff may not be available at many medical schools.

The greatest change in the curriculum with courses similar to the new pathway is seen in the preclinical faculty. Preclinical staff usually have busy schedules and may not be particularly well oriented to clinical matters. For example, teaching, say, the pharmacology of tetracycline in the traditional way is usually fairly easy for a preclinical pharmacologist with a related scientific interest. Less easy for (and possibly of less interest to) preclinical staff is dealing with a case study for the new pathway; such a case might start with the pharmacology of tetracyclines, pass through their therapeutic use in general, and end on a debate about whether oxytetracycline should be used as prophylaxis for traveller's diarrhoea in Mexico. Team teaching, with both preclinical and clinical staff present at each session, may be a feasible alternative, given the staff available at most medical schools.

It is true that the new pathway was oversubscribed in both pilot years. During the first pilot year, however, there was a sense amongst the "traditional" class that their colleagues in the new pathway were taking an extraordinary gamble with their medical education. During the second year this feeling persisted, but less strongly. I do not agree with Stella Lowry [pp 76-83] that "special arrangements that had been made for the new pathway students had caused resentment among other students, who felt that they were being treated like second class citizens."

Lastly, the success rate at Harvard in the national board examinations has always been extremely high (as it is at most American medical schools). These examinations are probably a poor instrument for measuring the quality of medical education because they concentrate on factual retention.

A W FOX

Raleigh, NC 27608,
USA

1 Lowry S. Making change happen. *BMJ* 1993;**306**:320-2.

Index